FOREWORD BY DAVE ASPREY

There's a reason that super hero movies are so popular. Just about every kid has dreamed of having a super power. As we grow up, adults teach us that those fantasies can't possibly happen, and we lose the dream.

Do you remember the super power you wanted when you were a kid? Did you believe it when adults said it was impossible? If you're like most people, you did, and you settled into the standard form of limited mediocrity that *most* of us know.

Except for a few stubborn people, those who keep the dream alive, and work to figure out how to make fantasies real. Because after all, powered flight was impossible... until one day someone did it.

The lesson here is that we believe things are impossible simply because we don't know how to do them, yet.

My name is Dave Asprey.

Because I somehow kept that curiosity alive, I was willing to spend over $1,000,000 working on my own biology to push the limits of what can do today, in the name of developing those super human powers we dream about.

To live beyond 180 years old (Matt and Wade also see themselves living well past 150). To have more energy, not less as I age. To have more control over my own biology and my own mind than most people believe is possible. And I've discovered that not only are these things possible, there is a rich community of people working on them.

This book shares many of the most effective biohacking techniques I've tested or discovered, plus many other ground-breaking concepts that have the power to at least improve your health, and maybe turn on more power than you think you have.

Biohacking is important. The media calls me the "Father of Biohacking" because I created the field, and it is the basis of several New York Times bestsellers I've written to share this vital knowledge.

Biohacking became one of 880 new words in the English language in 2018, and you'll find my name listed in the dictionary as a result! This is the knowledge that has fueled great changes in the field of health and nutrition over the last decade, along with my books, podcasts and the company I founded, Bulletproof.

Matt and Wade have been guests multiple times on the Bulletproof Radio podcast because they're a world of knowledge when it comes to nutrition, digestion and making yourself healthier. That's why I was happy to hear that they've compiled this knowledge into a book, and even happier to share a foreword.

In your hands, you hold a book that delivers the foundational building blocks to super-human health (which Matt and Wade call "BiOptimized Health"). If you just do half of the principles, process, strategies and technologies in this book, you can build extraordinary health, looks and performance. This easy to read knowledge stems from the methods that helped me go from an obese 300 lb man down to 200 lbs, boost my IQ by 20 points and become a better businessman, father and husband.

But it took me a million dollars and many years to "crack the code". I made many mistakes along the way. I overtrained. I followed diets that didn't work. Studying. Pushing. Staying up late. Getting an Ivy League MBA. Making $6 million before I turned twenty-seven. Unfortunately, I was overweight, exhausted and miserable, and I soon lost that $6 million.

However, it did let me spend what became more than $1 million to improve my biology at every level, from subcellular all the way to the highest spiritual levels I could find. Along the way, the first definition of biohacking came into focus as I honed in. It is the art and science of changing the environment inside and outside yourself so that you have full control of your own biology.

I've written New York Times bestsellers about the brain and willpower, interviewed almost a thousand researchers on consciousness and brains and biology Bulletproof Radio, earning 200 million downloads, and started a neuroscience facility for upgrading the human brain.

Based on those experiences, I feel confident stating that Matt and Wade have done a fabulous job synthesizing many cutting edge health breakthroughs into practical, bite-size pieces that you can implement in your life starting today. When you choose to follow their Biological Optimization Process, expect massive improvements across every spectrum of your health.

So many people experience unnecessary suffering physically and emotionally the way I did. With the knowledge in this book, you'll possess power to change that. It's up to you to make the decision, take responsibility and more importantly take action.

There's no reason for you not to wake up every day with a pep in your step and experience peak performance mentally... have the health and nervous-system to become ultra-resilient to modern stresses... and lose excess body fat and build lean muscle almost as a side effect. It's time to become BiOptimized!

Dave Asprey
CEO/Founder of Bulletproof
New York Times bestselling author of Head Strong And The Bulletproof Diet

TABLE OF CONTENTS

TABLE OF CONTENTS

TABLE OF CONTENTS

TABLE OF CONTENTS

INTRODUCTION

Why This Book Will Change Your Life

Imagine being able to wake up every day with a pep in your step and excitement to face the world.

Imagine keeping your mind and body decades younger than "the norm" and looking and feeling great well into your golden years.

Imagine being able to perform mentally at the highest levels for hours and hours without a single drop in energy... without any wavering in mental clarity... and without resorting to stimulants and other toxic chemicals.

Imagine a world where you can walk into virus and bacteria-infested environments with absolutely no fear, because you're confident your immune system can protect you.

In this book, you're going to discover what we consider the foundation for BiOptimized health.

Here are a few enlightening things you're going to learn:

- The truth about biological optimization—and why it goes beyond most health, fitness, and even modern "biohacking" advice.

- **The #1 nutrient for defeating stress and how to make your nervous system twice as resilient to outside stressors.**

- How dozens of dangerous toxins can "sneak" their way into healthy diets and lifestyles—and how to remove them for good.

- **The 5 most dangerous deficiencies, what causes them, and how to reverse them as rapidly as possible.**

- Why "reversing nutrient deficiency" is only HALF the battle (and the better way to think about nutrient uptake and performance).

- **Why nutrification goes beyond basic nutrition and helps you burn more fat, build muscle, and feel your best.**

- Why aging is OPTIONAL (and the 10 drivers of aging that you'll never hear mentioned in the mainstream media).

- **The secret to doubling your fat-burning "deep sleep" every night (and how to do this as affordably as possible).**

- The #1 thing you can do to turn your body into a 24/7 fat-burning machine—and why it's NOT calorie-cutting or cardio.

- **The most powerful form of exercise for weight-loss (hint: this is because it helps you detox and eliminate excess fluid and inches).**

- Not getting enough vitamin D? Most people don't—and it cripples their energy, immunity, and metabolism. Your vitamin D prescription...

- **How professional athletes, executives, celebrity trainers, and CEOs create their own "BiOptimization Blueprint"—and how you can, too...**

- The most powerful "BiOptimized" transformation any human can experience — in just 90 days or less.

Here's our mission at BiOptimizers:

> "End physical suffering by
> optimizing digestion and
> activating your BiOptimized health."

Your body is a miraculous machine. But in order to function at its best, you need to move towards biological optimization. That's what this book is about.

This book gives you THE CORE FUNDAMENTALS YOU NEED TO BECOME BIOLOGICALLY OPTIMIZED. If you do all the foundational basics in this book, you will experience extraordinary health, aesthetics, and performance.

This Blueprint is the culmination of 2-lifetimes of combined experiences helping others experience biological optimization. Plus, we are standing on the shoulders of our genius mentors.

We are happy to share everything we know with you inside this book. We hope it improves your life as much as it's improved the lives of those around us who apply its principles.

Armed with this information, you'll be able to experience a peak state of physical performance and super health... **We call it "BiOptimized Health": where you:**

- Look the way you really want.
- Perform mentally and physically at peak levels and...
- Maximize your lifespan and healthspan.

But be warned.

Once you start down this path you're going to be hooked on your new-found energy and vitality. You're going to feel so good that you won't want to stop.

Your health will continue to get stronger and stronger. Your energy will soar to new heights. Your metabolism will function the way Mother Nature intended it to. Your brain will "turn on" and you'll be amazed by your newfound drive and clarity.

We're confident this can happen for you because thousands of friends, family, and clients have experienced this with the same BiOptimization Blueprint you're reading right now.

For example...

- Wade's 67-year-old aunt was hit by a truck while driving her snowmobile. Her injuries included a broken ankle, fractured vertebrae, multiple lacerations, a serious concussion, and an assortment of other injuries. The doctors had little hope for her recovery. In just a few months, she was fully recovered and pain-free thanks to principles in this book.

- In just 16 weeks, we've helped a group of 40-year-old women get into bikini shape and compete in a fitness show, beating out women half their age.

- A burnt out 50 something hairstylist used these principles to detoxify his body from the countless chemicals he was exposed to over decades of working in the industry.
  Now over a decade later, he has more energy than he had in his twenties and travels internationally as a guest artist for one of the biggest hair product companies in the world.

- A 76-year-old man got off his antidepressants (that he was taking for decades), lost weight, found new love, and started a new business.

The bottom line is: we build healthy high-performance bodies from the inside out.

Are you ready for awesome health, a great looking body, and an optimized brain?

If you answered "YES" - read on...

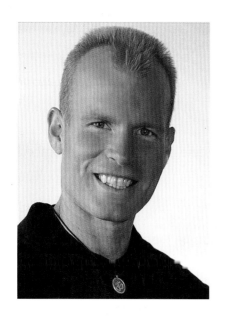

My name is Wade T Lightheart, advisor to the American Anti Cancer Institute, and 3-time all-natural bodybuilding champion. I'm also a certified sports nutrition advisor.

Despite my lousy genetics, I became one of the only vegetarians to ever compete in both the IFBB Mr. Universe contest and in the INBA Natural Mr. Olympia contest. Over my career, I won 13 bodybuilding titles in 5 different weight categories.

My passion and purpose for health came when I discovered the painful truth that doctors, drugs, and surgeries couldn't save my fit sister from dying of cancer at the age of 22.

I watched her get sick and go through four years of hell before she died. It tore my family apart. That activated a deep passion to understand what it means to be truly healthy because I didn't want a similar fate for myself.

So I went on to study exercise physiology and nutrition at the University of NB. I hired the best coaches in bodybuilding, I became a certified nutritionist, and more importantly, we put these ideas to the test. For the last 15 years, we've helped over 50,000 people achieve BiOptimized Health, and now it's your turn.

For many years I followed conventional bodybuilding protocols outlined by some of the most respected coaches and experts in the industry. But in the last years before the Mr. Universe competition, like many high-performance athletes, I was hiding a dark secret.

The long months of contest prep were excruciating. I could hardly sleep. My joints ached constantly. I was tired all the time and my muscles were so stiff and sore I could barely get out of bed in the morning. Matt said my brain function was in the "zombie zone".

The years of training, dieting, enzyme deficient diets, artificial sweeteners, and stimulants had taken their toll. I was burnt to a crisp.

After achieving my dream and competing at the Mr. Universe contest, I gained 42 pounds of fat and water in just 11 weeks. I went from Mr. Universe to Mr. Marshmallow. I felt like a walking nightmare.

I remember thinking to myself - *"There has to be a better way!"*

As destiny would have it, Matt and I were invited to a seminar held by a remarkable doctor who had reportedly healed himself and hundreds of patients from a variety of serious conditions.

The doctor was using a specialized protocol of medical-grade enzymes, probiotics, and live amino acids. Intrigued yet skeptical, we decided to investigate the doctor and his so-called "miracle protocols" for ourselves.

Over the course of two hours, his philosophy challenged almost every belief we had as a formally trained exercise physiologist, nutritionist, and athletes. **It blew our minds.**

My business partner, Matt Gallant, and I both decided to take a chance on his radical ideas and apply them, even though we have very different metabolisms and diet philosophies.

We used therapeutic dosages of enzymes and probiotics along with plant-based protein tokickstart the most amazing transformation of our lives. In 6 months I had completely healed my body, renewed my energy and vitality levels. I looked and felt better than I had in years.

After optimizing my body from the inside out, I returned to compete and shocked the bodybuilding community by winning a national championship with only 5 weeks of preparation. The best part is I felt amazing during the entire contest preparation with no rebound effects after the competition. I avoided the post-show weight gain and binging that most athletes experience.

This book reveals our best protocols and discoveries. If followed, they will aid you in achieving BiOptimized health, and give you the tools to successfully deal with the increasing toxicities in the world.

I am grateful to the many mentors, experts, and experiences that have led to this blueprint and sincerely believe in the benefits of these practices. After a few short weeks, you'll be very, very impressed with your new-found levels of health, vitality, and energy.

Wade T. Lightheart CSNA
President and Co-Founder of BiOptimizers
3 Time All Natural Bodybuilding Champion of Canada
Certified Sports Nutrition Advisor
Advisor to the American Cancer Institute

Who Are the Authors?

My name is Matt Gallant, kinesiologist, health researcher, and co-founder of BiOptimizers.

There are 3 experiences that formed my future around health.

The first was with my grandfather. **He prayed for death daily for the last 5 years of his life.**

He was the victim of a hit-and-run at the age of 75. It destroyed his hips and legs and he was never able to walk normally again. My father built an apartment for him in our home, so I got to spend time with him almost every day.

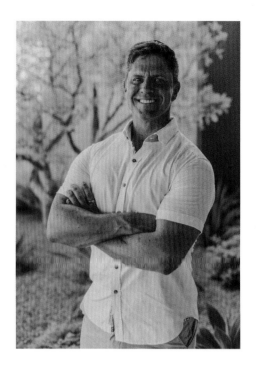

I saw his health decline over the last few years. For the last 5 years of his life, he was in so much pain that he prayed for death multiple times a day. The cocktail of painkillers and other pharmaceuticals didn't work anymore. It was a very emotional experience as a young teenager. This really showed me the value of health and maximizing healthspans (which we will talk about greatly in this book).

The second experience that marked me was going to the beach and seeing 2 bodybuilders. I was 16 years old and I wanted to look like that. That was the beginning of a passion for physical aesthetics. Since that time, I've been able to add over 60 lbs of lean muscle mass to my frame (despite having horrible genetics).

The 3rd was helping my best friend lose 191 lbs in 18 months when I was 19. Before this, he was a 20-year-old virgin who weighed 400 lbs and had never had a date.

I coached him for a year and a half and he became a new man. Not just physically, but mentally and emotionally. He got married shortly after. That impacted me so much that I knew this is what I wanted to do for a living. I wanted to help more people change not just how they look, but how they feel and help them upgrade themselves.

I got my bachelor's degrees in the science of physical activity and kinesiology and started helping hundreds of people.

I became one of the busiest trainers in Moncton and then in Vancouver, spending up to 80 hours a week in the gym. I have been blessed to train professional athletes in multiple sports and become close friends with many of the top minds in health and fitness.

At this time, I also became obsessed with hand-to-hand combat and self-defense. I started training with the legendary Christophe Clugston for many years. This was where I truly learned the keys and secrets to physical performance. His genius around optimizing and maximizing performance is truly world-class.

Then in 2001, I met Wade and we became close friends. We were both trainers and both shared a deep passion for health and fitness. In 2004, we decided to start a business together. That was the genesis of BiOptimizers.

We knew our destiny was to share this amazing information, products, and protocols with the world so that they can experience what BiOptimized health is.

Also around that same time, we met Dr. Michael O'Brien who taught us you could produce extraordinary results when you give the body the right "workers" and nutrients. We did his 90-day protocol and the rest his history. I got on his protocol and I dropped over 40 pounds and completely changed my health.

Over the next few years, we tested, optimized, and perfected the protocols with thousands of clients from around the world. The results were outstanding.

Our clinical experience led us to develop a whole suite of digestive solutions to truly fix and optimize your digestion and health. And that's why we created this Blueprint. Once you understand the 3 phases of nutrification, and how to optimize them you'll never look at food the same way.

My passion and purpose for helping others experience biological optimization have only gotten stronger in the last 2 decades.

Our goal is to keep innovating on every key component of health. We will not stop driving forward until we make biological optimization affordable and available to everyone on Earth.

Matt Gallant, Bsc. Sc. Of Phys. Act
CEO and Co-Founder of BiOptimizers
Kinesiologist

How to Read This Book

There are a few ways you can read this book. Choose the one that makes the most sense for you.

1 - Read from Cover to Cover

Of course, our suggestion is to read the book from cover to cover. There is a cohesive framework of biological optimization that will give you a solid understanding of how the body works.

When you understand the core problems and understand the solutions in-depth, you'll have more drive to take action. As trainers, we saw that people were far more successful long-term when they understood THE WHY. When you understand the biological reasons for struggle and success, you'll be far more willing to take action.

2 - Jump to the Solutions

If you want, you can jump right to the solutions section of the book and skip "The 4 Biological Enemies". The most important thing is to TAKE ACTION.

3 - Scan and Implement Powermoves

The book is loaded with Powermoves. The Powermoves are practical tips, hacks, and technologies that will improve your health, aesthetics, or performance. Just implementing these Powermoves will have a profound effect on your body.

4 - Jump to the Chapter You Need the Most Help With

If you're really pressed for time, just start by jumping to the chapter that you feel you need the most help with. If you're struggling with sleep, jump to that chapter. If you're struggling with digestion, jump to that section.

> The most important thing is to TAKE ACTION. TODAY.
> Implement the Powermoves into your daily life
> and turn them into HABITS.

Chapter 1

What is Biological Optimization?
(BiOptimization)

In this chapter, you will learn:

- **Why most approaches to health only lead you to average performance.**

- 3 secrets for realizing your full genetic potential for energy, vitality, and aesthetics.

- **The 4 biggest enemies that might stop your dreams and health goals.**

- And much more...

Biological optimization is a state where all of your body's functions operate in perfect harmony - a symphony of the factors flowing in optimal quantities and qualities. This means your hormones, lipids, blood sugar, liver enzymes, micronutrients, macronutrients, bio-workers, etc are all at optimal levels.

In fact, Our goal with this book is to help you become superhuman by helping you further along the BiOptimization Spectrum.

The Bioptimization Spectrum

FROM SICK TO SUPERHUMAN
BECOME BIOLOGICALLY OPTIMIZED

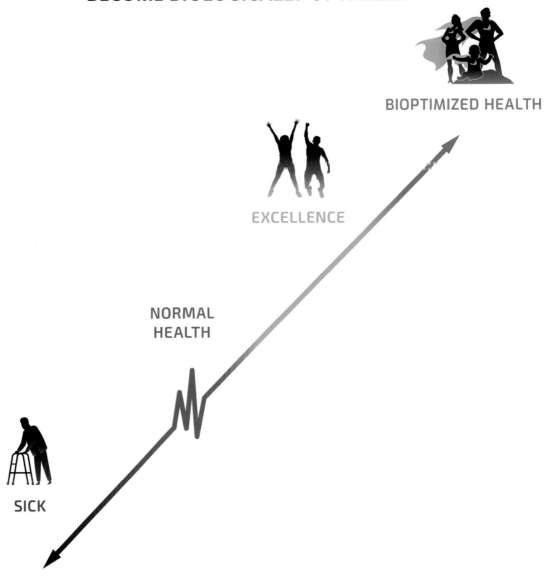

BIOPTIMIZED HEALTH

EXCELLENCE

NORMAL
HEALTH

SICK

There exist many definitions of health. The traditional medical definition of health is the "absence of disease."

While many people haven't been diagnosed with disease, most of us would agree that the lack of disease is not necessarily a good indicator of health, and it's certainly no indication of "super health" either.

Our definition of health goes beyond what many people consider "healthy." This state of health is far closer to our genetic potential as humans than mainstream medical science has led us to believe.

Everything from fitness to emotional well-being, immune system capacity, digestive health, brain function, and a host of other factors are all an integral part of health.

Until now, only a smart percentage of the population have experienced it and know how to maximize the various biological systems to optimal levels. This book is created to move you into the top end of the BiOptimization Spectrum.

The 3 Core Biological Optimization Processes

Every solution in this book falls into one of these 3 categories.

　　1 - Positive Stressors: the positive adaptations to biological stresses.

　　2 - Rejuvenation: the process of recovery and recuperation.

　　3 - Nutrification: the process of feeding the cells, organs, and body all of the nutrients they need
　　　　to function optimally.

By focusing on these 3 processes, you will maximize the 3 sides of the BiOptimization Triangle. You will kick aging in the butt. You will be in great shape and your performance will be at another level.

In a couple of decades, people will ask you "What are you doing? How do you have so much energy? How can I be in shape like you?"

Positive Stressors: What Doesn't Kill You Makes You Stronger

Positive stressors are what is known as hormesis in science. It's one of the most miraculous functions in the body. When we give the body the appropriate amount of stress, it will adapt in order to deal with that stress. Almost every biological optimization method functions because of this. It's the classic saying from Nietzsche "What doesn't kill you, makes you stronger." Of course, virtually too much of anything will kill us. This leads us to "What is the optimal dose?" That is a core principle of Biological Optimization and will discuss this throughout the book.

Rejuvenation

Rejuvenation is the process where the body heals itself. It's where recovery happens. Without maximizing your rejuvenation, your aesthetics, health, and performance will immediately suffer sharply. Over time, you'll experience dire consequences. The Powermoves found in the sleep and nervous system chapters are the keys to this.

Nutrification

Nutrification is a 3 phase process: consumption, conversion, and assimilation. First, you must consume high-quality foods that match your body's genetics, gut biome, and goals. Second, you must have the bio-workers (enzymes and probiotics) to break down and convert that food into their components: carbs into glycogen, protein into amino acids, and fats into fatty acids and glycerol. Finally, your body must assimilate those nutrients into either fuel or building blocks. We will go into great depth on how to optimize all 5 stages of digestion later in the book.

In order to succeed, we must do two things. First, we must eliminate or minimize the biggest enemies of biological optimization.

Second, we must maximize and optimize the factors that improve our health.

The 4 Biggest Enemies of Biological Optimization:

1 - Aging
2 - Stress
3 - Toxicity
4 - Nutrient deficiencies

We will go into depth on each one of these in the first part of the book.

The 7 Most Powerful Biological Optimizers:

1 - Nutrification
2 - High-quality sleep
3 - Lean muscle mass
4 - Movement
5 - Optimizing your nervous system
6 - Optimizing your brain
7 - Heliotherapy

The 7 Most Powerful Biological Optimizers

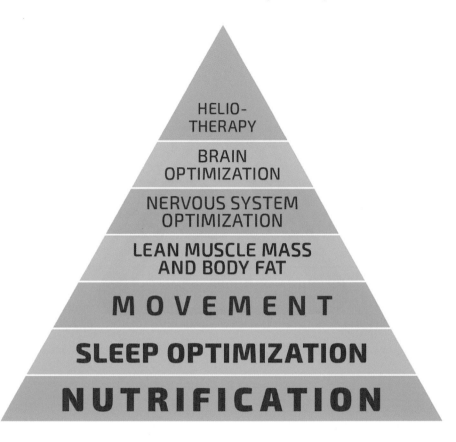

These are ordered based on the impact we believe they have on the body.

The foundational thing for great health is giving the body proper nutrients in the right quality and quantity. It's critical to optimize all 3 phases of the nutrification process, which we will talk about later in the book.

For many people, optimizing sleep is the #1 thing they can do to improve their overall health. High quality sleep impacts every aspect of your mind and body.

Movement, optimizing lean muscle mass, and lowering body fat not only have massive aesthetic results but as you will learn, they create incredible health-boosting benefits and help maximize your mental and physical performance.

In today's intense, fast-paced world, optimizing your nervous system and brain are critical for peak mental performance. If you want to know how to add decades to your mental prime, look no further.

And finally, heliotherapy is a significant health booster that amplifies the results of all the other biological optimizers.

We will cover all of these later in the book.

BiOptimization also means maximizing all 3 sides of the BiOptimization Triangle: aesthetics, performance, and health.

The Bioptimization Triangle

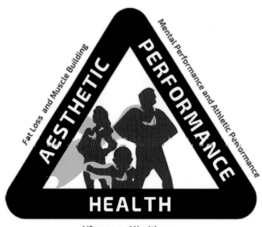

Optimizing Humans Since 2004

Aesthetics

Aesthetics is a highly personal goal. However, there are two truths that can't be denied:

> 1 - More lean muscle mass = better health and performance

> 2 - Less body fat = better health and performance (except if you're a sumo wrestler :-)

Adding lean body mass improves all 3 sides of the BiOptimization Triangle: aesthetics, performance, and health. Losing body fat also improves all 3 sides of the BiOptimization Triangle. [1] [2]

Our lean muscle tissue can account for more than 50% of our body mass. Muscles are vital from a metabolic perspective. It helps us control our glucose levels, use glucose as fuel, and reduce insulin resistance in type 2 diabetes. Loss of lean muscle mass contributes to poor health outcomes, fatigue, loss of function, disability, fall risk, frailty, and death.

[1] Srikanthan, P., & Karlamangla, A. S. (2014). Muscle mass index as a predictor of longevity in older adults. *The American journal of medicine*, 127(6), 547–553. https://doi.org/10.1016/j.amjmed.2014.02.007
[2] *People with low muscle strength more likely to die prematurely*. University of Michigan News. (2020). Retrieved 2 October 2020, from https://news.umich.edu/people-with-low-muscle-strength-more-likely-to-die-prematurely/.

Body fat isn't just aesthetically unpleasant, it's extremely unhealthy.[3] Fat cells cause inflammation. Willa Hsueh, M.D. states: "We did not know fat cells could instigate the inflammatory response," said principal investigator and Methodist Diabetes & Metabolism.

Some of the well-known and documented consequences of high body fat include:

- Type 2 diabetes.

- High blood pressure.

- Heart disease and strokes.

- Certain types of cancer.

- Sleep apnea.

- Osteoarthritis.

- Fatty liver disease.

- Kidney disease.

Optimizing Your Performance

Performance divides into 2 categories:

- Physical performance.

- Mental performance.

By following the advice in this book, you'll be able to achieve new levels of physical performance by optimizing your biology.

Physically: you'll be able to produce more energy, push yourself harder during training, and recover faster.

Mentally: you'll be able to work longer, focus better, rejuvenate your brain, and experience better overall brain function.

---

[3] Deng, T., Lyon, C. J., Minze, L. J., Lin, J., Zou, J., Liu, J. Z., Ren, Y., Yin, Z., Hamilton, D. J., Reardon, P. R., Sherman, V., Wang, H. Y., Phillips, K. J., Webb, P., Wong, S. T., Wang, R. F., & Hsueh, W. A. (2013). Class II major histocompatibility complex plays an essential role in obesity-induced adipose inflammation. *Cell metabolism*, 17(3), 411–422. https://doi.org/10.1016/j.cmet.2013.02.009

Optimizing Your Health

We define health as *LONGEVITY* and *VITALITY*.

Longevity can be broken down into lifespan and healthspan. We 100% believe that following the advice in this book can improve lifespan.

However, we KNOW with 100% certainty that following the advice in this book DOES improve healthspan. We define healthspan, as the length of the QUALITY of your health. Your healthspan is how long you remain healthy... How long you keep your vitality. You are in control of this. It's up to you to make a deep, unbreakable commitment to yourself to optimize and maximize your health.

In a typical ageing pattern, people's healthspan goes down dramatically in the last decade or two of their lives. By the time most people hit 60 years old, the loss of muscle mass compounded by years of being nutrient deficient combined with an overload of toxicity takes its toll. People become frail. Self-inflicted diseases emerge. It's a fast downward slope from here to decrepitness.

But, here's the great news: you've got the solution in your hands. You can live an incredible life filled with energy, vitality, and joy right until the day you pass on to the other side.

The Biological Optimization journey is a fun, rewarding adventure that changes how you feel. It transforms your emotional state. It gives you the drive to accomplish your dreams and goals. It changes your life.

Thanks to the ground-breaking discoveries in nutrition, brain physiology, biochemistry, and so on, we believe this state is attainable by almost everyone. Super health naturally occurs when all the right biological components are present and organs are functioning at their best.

However, we live in a complex, nutrient-deficient, and highly toxic world. This world can make it difficult to maintain BiOptimized health. Cellular functions and processes become compromised when the essential biological components are not present, or if there's an overload of toxic elements.

In chapter 4, you'll learn the various forms of toxicity around you. Simply being aware of the various chemicals and their sources will help you and your family avoid them.

In chapter 5, you'll discover how nutrient deficiency is the other major source of health problems today.

Those chapters are in the first part of this book which we call: *THE PROBLEM*.

In chapter 6 we will move into Part 2: *THE SOLUTION*.

The solution is *a process we call Biological Optimization*.

There are millions of biochemical and bioelectrical processes going on in your body at any given moment. Cells are growing, dying, and dividing constantly. Tens of thousands of enzymatic reactions are constantly happening in your blood, intestinal tract, muscles, and brain. In this book, you'll learn how to maximize and optimize the critical factors to boost your health.

Biological Optimization (*a.k.a. BiOptimization*), gives our cells, our organs, and our bodies all the resources they need to serve us in achieving super health, high performance, and awesome aesthetics.

This book will give you the key concepts you need to accomplish this and help you integrate them into your life.

We are happy to share with you the practices, principles, and products that have allowed us, and tens of thousands of our clients achieve remarkable levels of BiOptimized health.

This is the beginning of your journey to Biological Optimization.

The Biological Enemies

According to legendary football coach Don Shula, any time you wish to reach an objective, you have to realize that there are opposing forces working against you. The best strategy is to know these opposing forces and plan exactly how to overcome them to achieve your goal.

Likewise, in order for you to achieve super health and high performance, it's good to know the challenges and obstacles you must overcome.

Failure to recognize these challenges will accelerate aging and lower the quality of life in your later years. However, the Blueprint for BiOptimization has taken into account virtually all of these obstacles.

We have developed a step-by-step, easy to follow system that allows you to kick toxins' butts and address the fundamental causes of aging.

"The Biological Optimization Enemies" has some heavy science, but what's important is implementing the Powermoves mentioned throughout those chapters. By minimizing the Biological Enemies, you'll be able to truly minimize unnecessary aging and biological damage to your body.

Four Biological Enemies

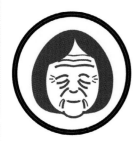

10 Aging
Drivers

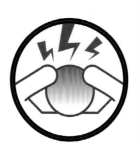

Stress

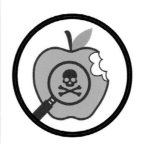

Toxins

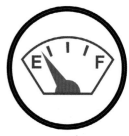

Deficiency

Chapter 2

Biological Enemy #1: The 10 Aging Drivers

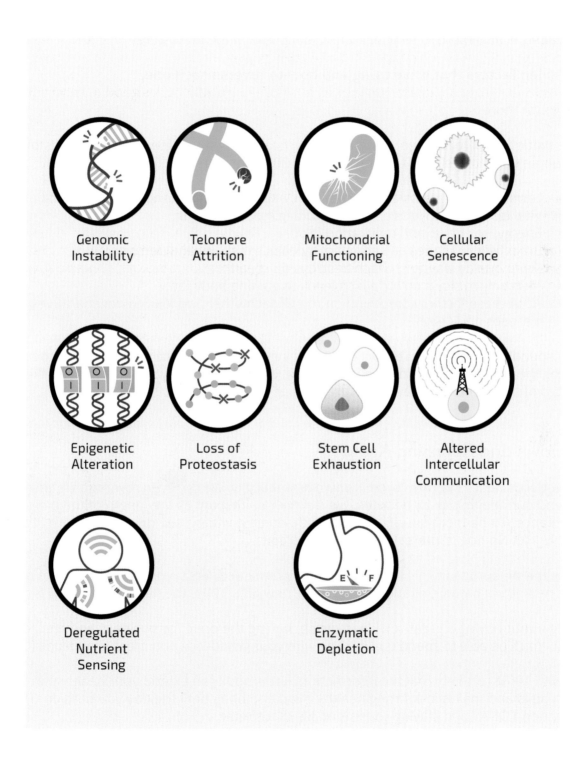

In this chapter, you will learn:

- **The NEW science of aging and why aging is a bigger threat than ever.**

- Why aging is also more reversible than at any point in human history.

- **10 hidden factors that drive aging and how to reverse each one.**

- And much more…

The biggest battle we all face when it comes to our healthspan and lifespan is aging. It's built into our DNA. The human body is designed to peak in its late 20s, procreate and then die.

- Hormones like testosterone, estrogen, and growth hormone begin declining.
- Vital lean muscle mass and strength begin deteriorating.
- Energy, sex drive, and motivation drop.
- Brain function fades and sometimes leads to senility and dementia.
- Sleep quality worsens, which destroys our health.
- Metabolism slows down, which leads to gaining body fat.
- All of these factors compound on top of each other and lead to degenerative diseases and death.

I know this sounds grim, but it's reality. The great news is: you've got the power to change this. By implementing the Powermoves throughout this book, you'll dramatically slow down all of these negative consequences of aging and even reverse a few.

Slowing Down and Reversing Aging

Thanks to modern science, we can slow this down dramatically. We can even reverse a lifetime of damage. We can extend our healthspan by decades. We define "healthspan" as the length of the biological body's high performance. To be more specific, it's strength, energy, vitality, sex drive, and more. It's the health quality of your life. No one is interested in being decrepit.

If you follow the blueprints in this book, barring any freak accidents, you'll avoid this fate and you can usher in the new youth paradigms such as: "80 is the new 50", "100 is the new 60" and "150 is the new 90".

We're talking about having a great sex life, dancing, having the drive for business and life… enjoying life to the fullest. You'll be able to spend quality time with your grand-kids and great-grand-kids (God willing).

We KNOW with 100% certainty that the information in this book can extend your healthspan by decades. Yes, you can build and maintain a strong healthy mind and body until the day you pass on. This requires you taking action TODAY and staying consistent. It's that simple.

Lifespan is how long we live. We have already made tremendous progress in this area in the last two centuries. And we're just getting started.

Normal aging vs. The Bioptimized lifestyle

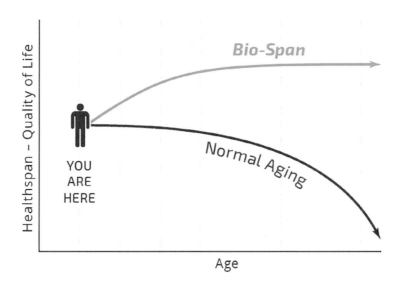

As you can see in the graph above, lifespan was stuck in the 30s and 40s for centuries. Now we're in the 70s and climbing. Contributors of this improvement came from advances in the medical system, antibiotics, improvements in economic prosperity, and more.

Eventually, advances in health technology will allow humans to live well into the 100s, maybe even 200s, and beyond. Some people are shooting for biological immortality.

We believe that the principles and methods in this book can extend lifespan dramatically. There is already tremendous scientific evidence showing major reductions in "All Cause Mortality" with several of the Powermoves that are in this book.

The biohackers and bioptimizers are a new breed of people. No long term study has been done with people who are stacking all of these methods. However, using simple induction and deduction, it stands to reason to think that we can live a much longer lifespan than our ancestors who didn't have this knowledge, health-tech, and supplements.

Powermove: Become Your Own Experiment

If you're going to wait for science to validate everything, you're always going to be 20-30 years behind. It takes decades for the practical applications from the geniuses living on the bleeding edge to make its way into double-blind studies. We are massive fans of research due to its ability to validate theories.

However, what really matters at the end of the day is
N = 1 and you're the 1. In other words, do your own experiments. Get professionals to help you: ASSESS, TEST, AND OPTIMIZE.

The 10 Aging Drivers

If we look at our DNA as software, we can state that it's designed to have an awesome user-experience until we get to our golden age. However, we have the power to upgrade the code thanks to epigenetics. If you implement the Biological Optimizers in this book, you'll positively upgrade your code and have a much better user-experience of life in your 80s, 90s, and beyond.

Warning: The next few pages are going to go deep into the science of aging. My suggestion, if it's too complex, just read it and focus on implementing the Powermoves in your life.[4]

1 - Genomic Instability
2 - Telomere Attrition
3 - Epigenetic Alteration
4 - Loss of Proteostasis
5 - Deregulated Nutrient Sensing
6 - Mitochondrial Functioning
7 - Cellular Senescence
8 - Stem Cell Exhaustion
9 - Altered Intercellular Communication
10 - Enzymatic Depletion

We're going to give a brief overview of each one of these 10 aging drivers. We could spend an entire book discussing aging however, we want to be pragmatic and practical. We're all about real-world results at BiOptimizers.

It's critical to note that the interlink and correlations between these aging drivers are very high. Some of them directly impact other aging drivers.

---

[4] López-Otín, C., Blasco, M. A., Partridge, L., Serrano, M., & Kroemer, G. (2013). The hallmarks of aging. *Cell*, 153(6), 1194–1217. https://doi.org/10.1016/j.cell.2013.05.039

Aging Driver #1: Genomic Instability

Imagine a brick building. If one brick in a wall crumbles, the wall will still hold. If a few more bricks get destroyed, the wall will still stand. But when enough bricks crumble, the wall will fall. The same thing applies to the building. A building can lose a non-structural wall and stay standing. However, if enough structural walls fall, the building will come tumbling down.

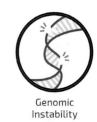

Genomic
Instability

In your body, your cells are like the bricks. Your organs are the walls and your body is the building. Now, imagine that each year certain cells' DNA becomes damaged. This then affects other cells and "the walls" will begin cracking. Eventually, the organs and body's systems will decline and in time, stop functioning. It would be time to get your Last Rights read. At that point, the "building falls", in other words, the body ceases to function. It's game over.

This is what happens over time as cells replicate themselves. Our DNA becomes damaged and these damaged cells impact the functioning of organs and create health issues.

What Damages Your DNA?

This is the key question. In the book "Biological DNA Sensor", Shimada and Co. break it down into 2 categories:

1. Endogenous damage caused by reactive oxygen species (ROS) that are derived from metabolic byproducts...

Powermove: Breath In 4th Phase Water Molecules

One of the most powerful technologies to deal with ROS damage is a high-tech machine that helps improve protein folding, which we'll discuss later in the chapter.

For more information, go here: *www.bioptimizers.com/blueprint-resources*

2. Exogenous damage caused by radiation (UV, X-ray, gamma), hydrolysis, toxins, and viruses.

We will cover toxins in a future chapter. Progressively eliminating toxins from your life and from your body will help minimize the damage.

Repair Enzymes

One of the answers to repairing the damage done by these factors is repair enzymes. Damaged DNA undergoes repair by a variety of repair enzymes such as endonucleases and exonucleases. These enzymes are typically found inside the mitochondria (which are the energy factories in your cells). This is one of the reasons to feed your body loads of enzymes. We believe the body can convert one type of enzyme into another and preserve your natural "enzyme bank account" (which we will cover in chapter 10).

Expect a lot of research, development, and breakthroughs in the next couple of decades in repair enzymes. Exercise is another key.

Exercise plays a role in maintaining genomic stability. In rodent models, aerobic exercise improves DNA repair mechanisms [5][6][7] Moreover, it increases DNA repair [8] and decreases the number of DNA/carcinogen entanglements up to 77%, related to aging. [9]

In other research, a six-month resistance training program with an elderly population led to improved resistance against genomic instability. [10]

We will discuss that in much greater depth in chapter 12.

[5] Gomez-Cabrera, M. C., Domenech, E., & Viña, J. (2008). Moderate exercise is an antioxidant: upregulation of antioxidant genes by training. *Free radical biology & medicine*, 44(2), 126–131. https://doi.org/10.1016/j.freeradbiomed.2007.02.001

[6] Leick, L., Lyngby, S. S., Wojtaszewski, J. F., & Pilegaard, H. (2010). PGC-1alpha is required for training-induced prevention of age-associated decline in mitochondrial enzymes in mouse skeletal muscle. *Experimental gerontology*, 45(5), 336–342. https://doi.org/10.1016/j.exger.2010.01.011

[7] Radák, Z., Naito, H., Kaneko, T., Tahara, S., Nakamoto, H., Takahashi, R., Cardozo-Pelaez, F., & Goto, S. (2002). Exercise training decreases DNA damage and increases DNA repair and resistance against oxidative stress of proteins in aged rat skeletal muscle. *Pflugers Archiv : European journal of physiology*, 445(2), 273–278. https://doi.org/10.1007/s00424-002-0918-6

[8] Cash, S. W., Beresford, S. A., Vaughan, T. L., Heagerty, P. J., Bernstein, L., White, E., & Neuhouser, M. L. (2014). Recent physical activity in relation to DNA damage and repair using the comet assay. *Journal of physical activity & health*, 11(4), 770–776. https://doi.org/10.1123/jpah.2012-0278

[9] Izzotti A. (2011). Genomic biomarkers and clinical outcomes of physical activity. *Annals of the New York Academy of Sciences*, 1229, 103–114. https://doi.org/10.1111/j.1749-6632.2011.06091.x

[10] Franzke, B., Halper, B., Hofmann, M., Oesen, S., Pierson, B., Cremer, A., Bacher, E., Fuchs, B., Baierl, A., Tosevska, A., Strasser, E. M., Wessner, B., Wagner, K. H., & Vienna Active Ageing Study Group (VAAS) (2015). The effect of six months of elastic band resistance training, nutritional supplementation or cognitive training on chromosomal damage in institutionalized elderly. *Experimental gerontology*, 65, 16–22. https://doi.org/10.1016/j.exger.2015.03.001

Aging Driver #2: Telomere Attrition

Telomeres are bits of DNA that are located at the ends of chromosomes. They help protect chromosomes from accidental fusion and DNA damage.

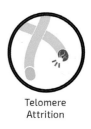

Telomere
Attrition

Just like making mixtapes with cassettes, copies become lower in quality as they are duplicated. Each time a cell divides, the DNA unwraps, and the information within is copied. Because of how cells divide, the telomere cannot be completely copied. A little bit gets cut off each time. It's believed that over time as it copies, the telomeres become shorter and shorter until they are gone.

When telomere sequences are fully lost, so is the cell's ability to replicate, rendering it less able to divide. Telomere exhaustion is thought to be one of the major contributors to cellular senescence, a.k.a. zombie cells.

Powermove: Track Your Telomeres

A simple test that you can do to track the length of your telomeres is called Teloyears. It's a simple, easy home test. We suggest doing it yearly to see if you're bioptimization lifestyle is having an impact. It's not uncommon to see major improvements in this arena.

Aging Driver #3: Epigenetic Alteration

Here's what's awesome about this one: you have control over this RIGHT NOW. As we stated earlier, this is your natural ability to rewrite your code.

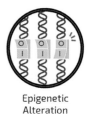

Epigenetic
Alteration

Prior to the understanding of epigenetics, everyone believed that genetics put everyone on a predestined fate. Your genes were your future. We bought into the dogma of genetic determinism. Now we know that's not the case.

Genetics certainly increase or decrease the probability of certain things happening. And yes, understanding your own genetics is one of the most empowering things you should do to maximize your health. Nutrigenomics is one of the most important parts of biological optimization. What that means is optimizing the dietary strategies, foods, and supplements you consume based on your genetics.

Here's the great news: you have an incredible level of control over your genetic expression.

Many of our genes are either: ON or OFF. In our pursuit of Biological Optimization, the goal is to turn on the good genes and turn off the bad ones. Almost all of the Powermoves in this book will help you do this.

There is a tremendous amount of research done in this area in terms of how our emotional and spiritual health affects these gene switches. One of the best books on the topic is, "The Genie In Your Genes" by Dawson Church.

Here's a passage from the book, *"The percentage by which genetic predisposition affects various conditions varies, but it is rarely 100%. The tools of our consciousness—including our beliefs, prayers, thoughts, intentions, and faith—often correlate much more strongly with our health, longevity, and happiness than our genes do. Larry Dossey, MD, observes,* **"Several studies show that what one thinks about one's health is one of the most accurate predictors of longevity ever discovered".**

You might think of DNA as version 1.0 of your code and epigenetics allows you to upgrade it. The key here is to understand that you're in far greater control of the commands your DNA receives than you might think.

How Epigenetic Alterations Accumulate

If we send "bad signals", meaning they aren't helping our health, these negative changes in the genome accumulate over time and have been correlated with the decline observed in aging cells.

Alterations to gene expression patterns are an important influencer of aging. Aging can cause changes to our epigenome, eventually compromising your cell's function. Remember that your cells are your body's building blocks, the bricks that create the walls.

An epigenome consists of a record of the chemical changes to your DNA; these changes can be passed down to your children via epigenetic inheritance.

Here's a shocking experiment that was done recently. Epigenetic experiments were done with roundworms. The epigenome was passed down 14 generations! Here's what this means for you, the epigenetics of your parents, grandparents, great-grand-parents, great-great-grandparents up to 14 generations back are part of your body today.

Inflammation is involved in epigenetic alterations. Studies show that caloric restriction slows the rate of these epigenetic changes. Metabolism and epigenetic alterations are closely linked with inflammation, creating a feedback loop leading to a vicious cycle. This is one of the main drivers of metabolic syndrome, which is one of the leading health problems today.

Metabolic syndrome is a cluster of conditions that are interlinked and usually happen together, increasing your risk of heart disease, stroke, and type 2 diabetes. These conditions include increased blood pressure, high blood sugar, excess body fat around the waist, and abnormal cholesterol or triglyceride levels. It's a vicious negative cycle from an epigenetic perspective.

The great news is, just taking action on the Powermoves in this book will help reverse this and start turning on the good gene switches.

Spirituality and Your Health

Does spirituality impact your health? The research says: ABSO-FREAKING-LUTELY.
Here are a few paragraphs from Dawson's "Genie In Your Genes" book:

"One such study was done by Thomas Oxman and his colleagues at the University of Texas Medical School. It examined the effects of social support and spiritual practice on patients undergoing heart surgery. It found that those with large amounts of both factors exhibited a mortality rate one-seventh of those who did not.[11]

Another was done at St. Luke's Medical Center in Chicago. It examined links between church attendance and physical health. The researchers found that patients who attended church regularly and had a strong faith practice were less likely to die and had stronger overall health.[12]

Larry Dossey, in "Prayer Is Good Medicine" says that there are over 1,200 scientific studies demonstrating the link between prayer and intention, and health and longevity. Meta-analyses in the Annals of Internal Medicine[13] and the Journal of Alternative and Complementary Medicine[14] have compiled the results of many studies and found that prayer, distant healing, and intentionality have significant effects on healing.

What about Spiritual Habits like helping others?

In her book The Energy Prescription, pharmacist Constance Grauds, RPh, describes one such study done in Michigan. It included a large sample, 2,700 men, and it studied them over a long period— nearly ten years. It found that the men who engaged in regular volunteer activities had death rates half of those who did not. She says that, "altruistic side effects include reduced stress; improved immune system functioning; a sense of joy, peace, and well-being; and even relief from physical and emotional pain. These effects tend to last long after the helping encounter, and...increase with the frequency of altruistic behavior." [15]

---

[11] Oxman, T. E., Freeman, D. H., Jr, & Manheimer, E. D. (1995). Lack of social participation or religious strength and comfort as risk factors for death after cardiac surgery in the elderly. *Psychosomatic medicine*, 57(1), 5–15. https://doi.org/10.1097/00006842-199501000-00002

[12] Powell, L. H., Shahabi, L., & Thoresen, C. E. (2003). Religion and spirituality. Linkages to physical health. *The American psychologist*, 58(1), 36–52. https://doi.org/10.1037/0003-066x.58.1.36

[13] Astin, J. A., Harkness, E., & Ernst, E. (2000). The efficacy of "distant healing": a systematic review of randomized trials. *Annals of internal medicine*, 132(11), 903–910. https://doi.org/10.7326/0003-4819-132-11-200006060-00009

[14] Jonas, W. (2001). The Middle Way: Realistic Randomized Controlled Trials for the Evaluation of Spiritual Healing. *The Journal Of Alternative And Complementary Medicine*, 7(1), 5-7. https://doi.org/10.1089/107555301300004466

[15] Musick, M. A., Herzog, A. R., & House, J. S. (1999). Volunteering and mortality among older adults: findings from a national sample. *The journals of gerontology. Series B, Psychological sciences and social sciences*, 54(3), S173–S180. https://doi.org/10.1093/geronb/54b.3.s173

Powermove: Be of Service

Make "giving your time" and spirituality a part of your life. Coach and mentor eager younger people FOR FREE. Go help a food shelter. Go clean up the beach, parks, and ditches. Meditate and pray.

Exercises Effect on Epigenetics

Physical exercise, both aerobic or resistance, can positively influence your epigenetics.

Endurance exercise training induces a number of adaptations in skeletal muscle, the most important of which is an increase in mitochondria with an improvement in respiratory capacity.

Some epigenetic modifications that possibly occur due to physical exercise can have a positive effect on restoring the genomic stability in cells with carcinogenic (cancer-causing) potential.[16]

There are numerous rapid mRNA and mitochondrial improvements to repeated high-intensity interval training sessions. Increases in mitochondrial proteins occurred within five days following three sessions of high-intensity interval training.[17]

Aging Driver #4: Loss of Proteostasis

The human body contains around 20,000 different proteins including 7,000 peptides. The maintenance and management of these proteins are called "proteostasis". These proteins and peptides do very specific functions in the body. When these functions decline in potency, it can lead to other health problems.

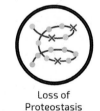

Loss of Proteostasis

Proteostasis ensures that the proteins and peptides are produced and folded appropriately before they travel to their target location in the body. Proteostasis stabilizes your proteins and keeps your cells properly functioning.[18] [19]

[16] Ntanasis-Stathopoulos, J., Tzanninis, J. G., Philippou, A., & Koutsilieris, M. (2013). Epigenetic regulation on gene expression induced by physical exercise. *Journal of musculoskeletal & neuronal interactions*, 13(2), 133–146.

[17] Perry, C. G., Lally, J., Holloway, G. P., Heigenhauser, G. J., Bonen, A., & Spriet, L. L. (2010). Repeated transient mRNA bursts precede increases in transcriptional and mitochondrial proteins during training in human skeletal muscle. *The Journal of physiology*, 588(Pt 23), 4795–4810. https://doi.org/10.1113/jphysiol.2010.199448

[18] Powers, E. T., Morimoto, R. I., Dillin, A., Kelly, J. W., & Balch, W. E. (2009). Biological and chemical approaches to diseases of proteostasis deficiency. *Annual review of biochemistry*, 78, 959–991. https://doi.org/10.1146/annurev.biochem.052308.114844

[19] Balch, W. E., Morimoto, R. I., Dillin, A., & Kelly, J. W. (2008). Adapting proteostasis for disease intervention. Science (New York, N.Y.), 319(5865), 916–919. https://doi.org/10.1126/science.1141448

Cellular proteostasis is key to ensuring successful development, healthy aging, resistance to environmental stresses, and to minimize the damage by pathogens such as viruses.

Molecular Chaperons: Heat Shock Proteins

One of the things that help with proteostasis is the activation of heat shock proteins (HSP). Sauna is one of the most amazing Powermoves anyone can integrate.

HSPs function as molecular chaperones that facilitate the synthesis and folding of proteins. These chaperones then act by protecting the proteins from further misfolding and promote either repair or degradation of damaged proteins. These proteins are what repairs your muscles and organs, creates critical neurotransmitters for optimal brain function.

Finland, who has a culture of using saunas, are the research leaders in saunas. The main study group is called the Kuopio Ischemic Heart Disease Risk Factor (KIHD) Study.

The KIHD findings revealed that men who used the sauna two to three times per week were 27 percent less likely to die from cardiovascular-related causes than men who didn't use the sauna.

Men who used the sauna roughly twice as often, about four to seven times per week, experienced roughly twice the benefits – and were 50 percent less likely to die from cardiovascular-related causes.

Even more impressive is, frequent sauna users were found to be 40 percent less likely to die from all causes of premature death.

The benefits on the brain were equally impressive. Men who used the sauna two to three times per week had a 66 percent lower risk of developing dementia and a 65 percent lower risk of developing Alzheimer's disease, compared to men who used the sauna only one time per week.[20]

Dr. Rhonda Patrick does a great job breaking down the research. Her website is *www.foundmyfitness.com*

Powermove: Sweat in the Sauna

This Powermove can easily be achieved by spending 15 to 30 minutes in a hot sauna 3-6 times a week. Two to three times a week have a massive impact on your overall health. Four to seven times increases the benefits even more.

---

[20] Kukkonen-Harjula, K., & Kauppinen, K. (2006). Health effects and risks of sauna bathing. *International journal of circumpolar health,* 65(3), 195–205. https://doi.org/10.3402/ijch.v65i3.18102

Aging Driver #5: Deregulated Nutrient Sensing

Your body has built-in sensors to detect certain nutrients. These sensors become less functional as we age. The four associated key protein groups are IGF-1, mTOR, sirtuins, and AMPK. We call these proteins "nutrient-sensing" because various nutrient levels influence their activity.

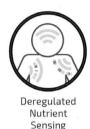

Deregulated Nutrient Sensing

The GH/IGF Axis

IGF is an acronym for "insulin-like growth factors". IGF-1 is primarily controlled by GH levels in the body. They operate on an axis, meaning they influence each other.

IGF-1 is considered to be the most anabolic hormone in the body by many bodybuilders.[21] [22] IGF-1 is often stacked with growth hormone and anabolic steroids to enhance the anabolic effects.

The concerns with IGF-1 are that they stimulate growth in all the tissues in the body including tumors. In short, IGF is a potent enhancer of aesthetics, performance, and healthspan. However, lifespan should be factored. That's why we believe that to maximize all sides of the BiOptimization Triangle, it's wise to cycle between anabolic phases and autophagic phases. More on this in a minute.

mTOR: The Anabolic Activator

mTOR is a champion regulator of anabolic metabolism, the process of building new proteins and tissues. In this way, it functions similar to IGF. At any given moment, the metabolism is either breaking down old parts (autophagy/catabolism) or building new ones (growth/anabolism). Both mTOR and the IGF are part of the anabolic side of metabolism.

Powermove: Consume Leucine Before Each Meal

The mTOR activating amino acid, Leucine, has been shown in research to be extremely effective at activating mTOR. Three to seven grams per meal will improve anabolism.

21 Anderson, L. J., Tamayose, J. M., & Garcia, J. M. (2018). Use of growth hormone, IGF-I, and insulin for anabolic purpose: Pharmacological basis, methods of detection, and adverse effects. *Molecular and cellular endocrinology*, 464, 65–74. https://doi.org/10.1016/j.mce.2017.06.010

22 Guha, N., Cowan, D. A., Sönksen, P. H., & Holt, R. I. (2013). Insulin-like growth factor-I (IGF-I) misuse in athletes and potential methods for detection. *Analytical and bioanalytical chemistry*, 405(30), 9669–9683. https://doi.org/10.1007/s00216-013-7229-y

This is a powerful tool for anyone seeking to improve lean muscle mass and athletic performance. Leucine is why whey protein has been shown to be more anabolic than most other proteins. Whey protein contains about 10% leucine levels.

For people wanting to avoid dairy, we suggest consuming 5 grams of leucine with their meals to improve anabolic response. Another alternative is 1 gram of HMB 30 minutes before a meal.

Sirtuins

The sirtuin genes are believed to be one of the most promising longevity genes. There are seven sirtuins in mammals, SIRT1 to SIRT7, and they are made by almost every cell in the body.[23]

David Sinclair is one of the world's leading anti-aging researchers and preeminent experts in sirtuins. *"These critical epigenetic regulators sit at the very top of cellular control systems, controlling our reproduction and our DNA repair."*

There is a strong relationship between NAD and sirtuins. The decline of NAD as we age, and the resulting decline in sirtuin activity, is believed to be one of the main reasons why our bodies develop diseases when we are old but not when we are young.[24]

Sirtuins can reduce inflammation that drives diseases such as atherosclerosis, metabolic disorders, ulcerative colitis, arthritis, and asthma.

They also help make mitochondria stronger. In studies on mice, activating the sirtuins can improve DNA repair, boost memory, increase exercise endurance, and help the mice stay thin, regardless of what they eat.

Exercise is one of the main ways to boost sirtuin expression.

AMPK

AMPK plays a role in cellular energy homeostasis, largely to activate glucose and fatty acid uptake and oxidation when cellular energy is low. Basically, when you're fasting or low on calories, AMPK goes up.

---

[23] Frye R. A. (2000). Phylogenetic classification of prokaryotic and eukaryotic Sir2-like proteins. *Biochemical and biophysical research communications*, 273(2), 793–798. https://doi.org/10.1006/bbrc.2000.3000
[24] Sinclair, D. (2019). *Lifespan*. Thorsons.

It just needs to be done.

AMPK is basically a sensor of fasted or calorie-restricted states and catabolism.[25] Catabolism uses energy to break down.[26] By doing so, AMPK helps regulate metabolism.[27]

Powermove: Fasting

Fasting is one of the most powerful ways to improve overall health. There are many forms of fasting. Starting with a 1-day fast is an easy place to start. Doing a 3-day fast once a month or once a quarter has been shown to have powerful regenerative effects on the immune system.[28]

Wade and Matt love incorporating fasting every week. They've had tremendous success doing alternate-day fasting. The more you fast, the easier it gets.

Intermittent fasting has also become a popular trend in the last few years. You can start with a 16-8 window (16 hours of fasting and 8 hours of eating). Then you can move to 20-4 (20 hours of eating and 4 hours of fasting) and some people move to OMAD (one meal a day).

Like sirtuins, higher activity of AMPK has longevity-promoting effects. Metformin, a diabetes drug that appears to have a life extension effect, activates AMPK in mice and worms.[29]

It is believed that lower AMPK sensitivity can lead to cellular inflammation, reduced autophagy, metabolic syndrome, and more fat disposition.[30]

In summary, there are four key proteins involved in nutrient sensing that might be key contributors to aging. Turning down the pathways of the first two, IGF-1 and mTOR, promotes longevity. In states of calorie and protein abundance, these two increase anabolism.

[25] López-Otín, C., Blasco, M. A., Partridge, L., Serrano, M., & Kroemer, G. (2013). The hallmarks of aging. *Cell*, 153(6), 1194–1217. https://doi.org/10.1016/j.cell.2013.05.039

[26] Salminen, A., & Kaarniranta, K. (2012). AMP-activated protein kinase (AMPK) controls the aging process via an integrated signaling network. *Ageing research reviews*, 11(2), 230–241. https://doi.org/10.1016/j.arr.2011.12.005

[27] López-Otín, C., Blasco, M. A., Partridge, L., Serrano, M., & Kroemer, G. (2013). The hallmarks of aging. *Cell*, 153(6), 1194–1217. https://doi.org/10.1016/j.cell.2013.05.039

[28] Cheng, C. W., Adams, G. B., Perin, L., Wei, M., Zhou, X., Lam, B. S., Da Sacco, S., Mirisola, M., Quinn, D. I., Dorff, T. B., Kopchick, J. J., & Longo, V. D. (2014). Prolonged fasting reduces IGF-1/PKA to promote hematopoietic-stem-cell-based regeneration and reverse immunosuppression. *Cell stem cell*, 14(6), 810–823. https://doi.org/10.1016/j.stem.2014.04.014

[29] López-Otín, C., Blasco, M. A., Partridge, L., Serrano, M., & Kroemer, G. (2013). The hallmarks of aging. *Cell*, 153(6), 1194–1217. https://doi.org/10.1016/j.cell.2013.05.039

[30] Salminen A, Kaarniranta K. AMP-activated protein kinase (AMPK) controls the aging process via an integrated signaling network. *Ageing Res Rev.* 2012;11(2):230-241. doi:10.1016/j.arr.2011.12.005

Conversely, AMPK and sirtuins increase with nutrient scarcity. They are believed to help with longevity. They work to promote autophagy.[31] Autophagy is the body's way of cleaning out cellular damage in order to regenerate newer, healthier cells, according to Priya Khorana, Ph.D., in nutrition education from Columbia University. "Auto" means self and "phagy" means eat. So the literal meaning of autophagy is "self-eating." [32]

Multiple studies have demonstrated that caloric restriction can slow the aging decline.[33]

On a cellular level, pathways fine-tuning metabolic regulation, such as the mTOR or insulin pathway, have also been linked to increased healthspan and lifespan.[34]

 ## Powermove: Cycle Between Autophagic and Anabolic Phases

To get the best of both worlds, healthspan and lifespan, cycle between periods of anabolism and autophagy. During the anabolic periods, you'll get to enjoy more foods, add on muscle mass, and get stronger. These are fantastic to improve performance and healthspan.

Then cycle to an autophagic weight-loss cycle and fast, clean the body on a cellular level, burn body fat, activate AMPK and sirtuins. What that looks like in the real world is, you might spend 4-8 weeks on a higher calorie muscle-building cycle.

Then, drop calories, incorporate fasting, and lose body fat. This is the strategy Matt has been doing for the last 5 years and has been able to lose 3-8 lbs of body fat and gain 3-8 lbs of lean muscle mass per year. It's also one of the best strategies for improving your aesthetics.

Matt and Wade have also used a weekly cycling strategy that has produced amazing results. They fast 3 days a week on alternate days, for example: Monday, Wednesday, and Friday. Have 2 days of maintenance level calories with 3 meals: Tuesday and Thursday. And then two days of high-carb, high-calorie days to boost up metabolism and anabolism. Matt dropped 26 lbs in the first 9 weeks. Wade dropped 20 lbs in 8 weeks.

[31] López-Otín, C., Blasco, M. A., Partridge, L., Serrano, M., & Kroemer, G. (2013). The hallmarks of aging. *Cell*, 153(6), 1194–1217. https://doi.org/10.1016/j.cell.2013.05.039

[32] *Autophagy: Definition, Diet, Fasting, Cancer, Benefits, and More.* Healthline. (2020). Retrieved 2 October 2020, from https://www.healthline.com/health/autophagy.

[33] Mitchell, S. J., Madrigal-Matute, J., Scheibye-Knudsen, M., Fang, E., Aon, M., González-Reyes, J. A., Cortassa, S., Kaushik, S., Gonzalez-Freire, M., Patel, B., Wahl, D., Ali, A., Calvo-Rubio, M., Burón, M. I., Guiterrez, V., Ward, T. M., Palacios, H. H., Cai, H., Frederick, D. W., Hine, C., … de Cabo, R. (2016). Effects of Sex, Strain, and Energy Intake on Hallmarks of Aging in Mice. *Cell metabolism*, 23(6), 1093–1112. https://doi.org/10.1016/j.cmet.2016.05.027

[34] Harrison, D. E., Strong, R., Sharp, Z. D., Nelson, J. F., Astle, C. M., Flurkey, K., Nadon, N. L., Wilkinson, J. E., Frenkel, K., Carter, C. S., Pahor, M., Javors, M. A., Fernandez, E., & Miller, R. A. (2009). Rapamycin fed late in life extends lifespan in genetically heterogeneous mice. *Nature*, 460(7253), 392–395. https://doi.org/10.1038/nature08221

Aging Driver #6: Mitochondrial Functioning

Mitochondria are the little energy factories inside your cells. They produce ATP which is what your body uses for fuel.

The problem is that mitochondria die and become weaker with age unless you stress them the positive stressors and feed them properly.

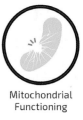

Mitochondrial Functioning

A decline in mitochondrial quality and activity has been associated with normal aging[35] and correlated with the development of a wide range of age-related diseases. Here, we review the evidence that a decline in mitochondria function contributes to aging.

Powermove: HIIT and mitochondria

One of the most powerful ways to boost mitochondria is high-intensity interval training. In a few weeks of interval bike training.[36] It's a wise move to incorporate 1 or 2 HIIT workouts in a week in your lifestyle.

Mitochondria as Regulators of Stem Cell Function

It is believed that mitochondria might be an important regulator of stem cells. A decline in adult stem cell function is thought to contribute to various aspects of aging.[37]

Mitochondria and Cellular Senescence

We will discuss cellular senescence in-depth in a moment, but it is believed that mitochondria play a role

[35] ROCKSTEIN, M., & BRANDT, K. F. (1963). Enzyme changes in flight muscle correlated with aging and flight ability in the male housefly. *Science (New York, N.Y.)*, 139(3559), 1049–1051. https://doi.org/10.1126/science.139.3559.1049
[36] Robinson, M. M., Dasari, S., Konopka, A. R., Johnson, M. L., Manjunatha, S., Esponda, R. R., Carter, R. E., Lanza, I. R., & Nair, K. S. (2017). Enhanced Protein Translation Underlies Improved Metabolic and Physical Adaptations to Different Exercise Training Modes in Young and Old Humans. *Cell metabolism*, 25(3), 581–592. https://doi.org/10.1016/j.cmet.2017.02.009
[37] López-Otín, C., Blasco, M. A., Partridge, L., Serrano, M., & Kroemer, G. (2013). The hallmarks of aging. *Cell*, 153(6), 1194–1217. https://doi.org/10.1016/j.cell.2013.05.039

in managing cellular senescence.[38]

Powermove: Cold Therapy and Mitochondria

There is evidence that cold therapy improves mitochondrial health through a process known as "mitochondrial biogenesis," or in other words, by producing more of them.[39]

Boost your mitochondria by ending your hot showers with 30 seconds of water as cold as you can tolerate it. Even 30 - 90 seconds of cold water can have profound effects according to a study in *PLoS One*.[40] For those wanting to take it further, two bags of ice in a bathtub filled with water is a simple ice bath hack.

Mitochondria and Inflammation [41]

One of the drivers of aging is the development of a low-grade, chronic inflammatory state often deemed 'inflammaging'. It's wise to do blood tests and look at circulating inflammatory biomarkers such as IL-6 and C-reactive protein. There seems to be a strong connection between mitochondrial function and inflammation.[42]

[38] Quijano, C., Cao, L., Fergusson, M. M., Romero, H., Liu, J., Gutkind, S., Rovira, I. I., Mohney, R. P., Karoly, E. D., & Finkel, T. (2012). Oncogene-induced senescence results in marked metabolic and bioenergetic alterations. *Cell cycle (Georgetown, Tex.)*, 11(7), 1383–1392. https://doi.org/10.4161/cc.19800

[39] Chung, N., Park, J., & Lim, K. (2017). The effects of exercise and cold exposure on mitochondrial biogenesis in skeletal muscle and white adipose tissue. *Journal of exercise nutrition & biochemistry*, 21(2), 39–47. https://doi.org/10.20463/jenb.2017.0020

[40] Buijze, G. A., Sierevelt, I. N., van der Heijden, B., Dijkgraaf, M. G., & Frings-Dresen, M. (2018). Correction: The Effect of Cold Showering on Health and Work: A Randomized Controlled Trial. *PloS one*, 13(8), e0201978. https://doi.org/10.1371/journal.pone.0201978

[41] Chung, N., Park, J., & Lim, K. (2017). The effects of exercise and cold exposure on mitochondrial biogenesis in skeletal muscle and white adipose tissue. *Journal of exercise nutrition & biochemistry*, 21(2), 39–47. https://doi.org/10.20463/jenb.2017.0020

[42] Franceschi, C., Bonafè, M., Valensin, S., Olivieri, F., De Luca, M., Ottaviani, E., & De Benedictis, G. (2000). Inflamm-aging. An evolutionary perspective on immunosenescence. *Annals of the New York Academy of Sciences*, 908, 244–254. https://doi.org/10.1111/j.1749-6632.2000.tb06651.x

Powermove: kApex

Take 3-5 capsules of kApex upon awakening. kApex is a supplement formula designed to help transport more essential fatty acids to the mitochondria. And make the mitochondria stronger. It helps activate AMPK and can supply 6-10 hours of constant energy without taxing adrenal glands.

Aging Driver #7: Cellular Senescence

"Zombie cells", known as cellular senescence are the decrepit cells in your body that create chaos.

Cellular senescence is when cells can no longer divide. In their groundbreaking experiments during the early 1960s, Leonard Hayflick and Paul Moorhead found that normal human cells in culture reach a maximum of approximately 50 cell population doublings before becoming senescent.[43][44][45]

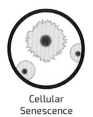

Cellular
Senescence

The inability of **senescent cells** to proliferate can impair tissue regeneration after injury, causing prolonged or permanent tissue damage with age. Although senescent cells can no longer replicate, they remain metabolically active and become pro-inflammatory.

Powermove: Eliminate Senescent Cells

Metformin is one of the most well-researched and promising anti-aging drugs currently known. It is commonly used for managing blood sugar with diabetes. Metformin fights

[43] Collado, M., Blasco, M. A., & Serrano, M. (2007). Cellular senescence in cancer and aging. *Cell*, 130(2), 223–233. https://doi.org/10.1016/j.cell.2007.07.003
[44] Hayat, M. (2014). *Tumor Dormancy, Quiescence, and Senescence, Vol. 3.* Springer Netherlands.
[45] Tollefsbol, T. (2010). *Epigenetics of aging. Springer.*

cancer[46] [47] and increases lifespan in both rodents and human cells[48] [49] by reducing senescence.

The one caveat is that metformin depletes vitamin B12, so make sure to add some methylated b-12 in your supplement stack. You may also want to cycle on and off of metformin.[50] It is wise in general to cycle on and off of supplements. Consult with your doctor.

Fisetin is a natural polyphenol found in seaweed and strawberries. Fisetin destroys senescent cells and increases lifespan by 10% in rodents.[51]

Aging Driver #8: Stem Cell Exhaustion

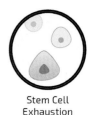

Stem Cell
Exhaustion

Stem cells are special human cells that are able to transform into many different cell types. This can range from muscle cells to brain cells.

Stem cells provide new cells for the body as it grows, and replace specialized cells that are damaged or lost. They have two attributes that make them do this:

- They can divide over and over again to produce new cells.

- As they divide, they can transform into the other types of cells that make up the body.

Stem cells are one of the most important cellular repair systems in your body. As we get older, stem cells

46 Hosono, K., Endo, H., Takahashi, H., Sugiyama, M., Sakai, E., Uchiyama, T., Suzuki, K., Iida, H., Sakamoto, Y., Yoneda, K., Koide, T., Tokoro, C., Abe, Y., Inamori, M., Nakagama, H., & Nakajima, A. (2010). Metformin suppresses colorectal aberrant crypt foci in a short-term clinical trial. *Cancer prevention research (Philadelphia, Pa.), 3*(9), 1077–1083. https://doi.org/10.1158/1940-6207.CAPR-10-0186

47 Memmott, R. M., Mercado, J. R., Maier, C. R., Kawabata, S., Fox, S. D., & Dennis, P. A. (2010). Metformin prevents tobacco carcinogen--induced lung tumorigenesis. *Cancer prevention research (Philadelphia, Pa.), 3*(9), 1066–1076. https://doi.org/10.1158/1940-6207.CAPR-10-0055

48 Fang, J., Yang, J., Wu, X., Zhang, G., Li, T., Wang, X., Zhang, H., Wang, C. C., Liu, G. H., & Wang, L. (2018). Metformin alleviates human cellular aging by upregulating the endoplasmic reticulum glutathione peroxidase 7. *Aging cell, 17*(4), e12765. https://doi.org/10.1111/acel.12765

49 Martin-Montalvo, A., Mercken, E. M., Mitchell, S. J., Palacios, H. H., Mote, P. L., Scheibye-Knudsen, M., Gomes, A. P., Ward, T. M., Minor, R. K., Blouin, M. J., Schwab, M., Pollak, M., Zhang, Y., Yu, Y., Becker, K. G., Bohr, V. A., Ingram, D. K., Sinclair, D. A., Wolf, N. S., Spindler, S. R., ... de Cabo, R. (2013). Metformin improves healthspan and lifespan in mice. *Nature communications, 4,* 2192. https://doi.org/10.1038/ncomms3192

50 Reinstatler, L., Qi, Y. P., Williamson, R. S., Garn, J. V., & Oakley, G. P., Jr (2012). Association of biochemical B12 deficiency with metformin therapy and vitamin B12 supplements: the National Health and Nutrition Examination Survey, 1999-2006. *Diabetes care, 35*(2), 327–333. https://doi.org/10.2337/dc11-1582

51 Yousefzadeh, M. J., Zhu, Y., McGowan, S. J., Angelini, L., Fuhrmann-Stroissnigg, H., Xu, M., Ling, Y. Y., Melos, K. I., Pirtskhalava, T., Inman, C. L., McGuckian, C., Wade, E. A., Kato, J. I., Grassi, D., Wentworth, M., Burd, C. E., Arriaga, E. A., Ladiges, W. L., Tchkonia, T., Kirkland, J. L., ... Niedernhofer, L. J. (2018). Fisetin is a senotherapeutic that extends health and lifespan. *EBioMedicine, 36,* 18–28. https://doi.org/10.1016/j.ebiom.2018.09.015

become depleted. **Stem cell exhaustion** is observed in virtually all tissues.[52]

As we get older, the activity of our stem cells slowly decreases for a few reasons. For instance, senescent cells constantly secrete pro-inflammatory, immunosuppressive chemicals, which reduces stem cell activity. These contribute to immune senescence and loss of tissue regeneration. As we've said a few times, these 10 aging drivers are interlinked and correlated.

Powermove: Boost Stem Cells Naturally

There are a few things you can do to boost stem cells naturally:

1 -   Intermittent fasting is a great strategy for improving natural stem cells.

2 -   Get great sleep (read chapter 11). Research has shown that lack of sleep or insomnia is very detrimental to stem cell function in the body. A reduction of night sleep to 4 hours (instead of 8) decreases the ability of stem cells to migrate by nearly 50% while proper 7-8 hour sleep cycles do the opposite and renew the quantitative and qualitative indices of circulating stem cells.

3 -   Although the work is preliminary,[53] there are data that the polyphenols and

        antioxidants found in blueberries, green tea, pomegranates, goji berries,[54] and even spirulina can increase circulating bone-marrow-derived stem cells.

4 -   Research[55] indicates that the response to bouts of acute exercise includes increases in stem cells in the circulation.

[52] Ren, R., Ocampo, A., Liu, G. H., & Izpisua Belmonte, J. C. (2017). Regulation of Stem Cell Aging by Metabolism and Epigenetics. *Cell metabolism*, 26(3), 460–474. https://doi.org/10.1016/j.cmet.2017.07.019

[53] Zhang, J., Lazarenko, O. P., Blackburn, M. L., Shankar, K., Badger, T. M., Ronis, M. J., & Chen, J. R. (2011). Feeding blueberry diets in early life prevent senescence of osteoblasts and bone loss in ovariectomized adult female rats. *PloS one*, 6(9), e24486. https://doi.org/10.1371/journal.pone.0024486

[54] Mikirova, N. A., Jackson, J. A., Hunninghake, R., Kenyon, J., Chan, K. W., Swindlehurst, C. A., Minev, B., Patel, A. N., Murphy, M. P., Smith, L., Ramos, F., Ichim, T. E., & Riordan, N. H. (2010). Nutraceutical augmentation of circulating endothelial progenitor cells and hematopoietic stem cells in human subjects. *Journal of translational medicine*, 8, 34. https://doi.org/10.1186/1479-5876-8-34

[55] Emmons, R., Niemiro, G. M., Owolabi, O., & De Lisio, M. (2016). Acute exercise mobilizes hematopoietic stem **and progenitor** cells and alters the mesenchymal stromal cell secretome. *Journal of applied physiology (Bethesda, Md. : 1985)*, 120(6), 624–632. https://doi.org/10.1152/japplphysiol.00925.2015

Stem cells are also not immune to direct damage and destruction: telomere shortening, for instance, can lead to stem cells losing function[56] and becoming senescent.[57] And their DNA can slowly mutate to the point of causing senescence or cancer.[58]

A reduction in stem cell activity can lead to many diseases and general issues, such as immunosuppression through reduced production of bacteria-killing and virus-killing white blood cells,[59] muscle loss, frailty, and the weakening of bones.[60] [61]

Powermove: Stem Cell Therapy

One of the most promising areas of research is stem cells. Based on early data, and anecdotal evidence it might be one of the most powerful anti-aging treatments available.

The downsides include: traveling to foreign locations because many governments are not allowing certain types of treatments, the unknown risks of the procedures (which seems low based on current data), and the costs. However, for those with the money, this could be a fantastic investment in healthspan and lifespan. Expect the price to drop rapidly over time.

---

[56] Hiyama, E., & Hiyama, K. (2007). Telomere and telomerase in stem cells. *British journal of cancer,* 96(7), 1020–1024. https://doi.org/10.1038/sj.bjc.6603671
[57] Herbig, U., Jobling, W. A., Chen, B. P., Chen, D. J., & Sedivy, J. M. (2004). Telomere shortening triggers senescence of human cells through a pathway involving ATM, p53, and p21(CIP1), but not p16(INK4a). *Molecular cell,* 14(4), 501–513. https://doi.org/10.1016/s1097-2765(04)00256-4
[58] Adams, P. D., Jasper, H., & Rudolph, K. L. (2015). Aging-Induced Stem Cell Mutations as Drivers for Disease and Cancer. *Cell stem cell,* 16(6), 601–612. https://doi.org/10.1016/j.stem.2015.05.002
[59] Warren, L. A., & Rossi, D. J. (2009). Stem cells and aging in the hematopoietic system. *Mechanisms of ageing and development,* 130(1-2), 46–53. https://doi.org/10.1016/j.mad.2008.03.010
[60] López-Otín, C., Blasco, M. A., Partridge, L., Serrano, M., & Kroemer, G. (2013). The hallmarks of aging. *Cell,* 153(6), 1194–1217. https://doi.org/10.1016/j.cell.2013.05.039
[61] Ahmed, A. S., Sheng, M. H., Wasnik, S., Baylink, D. J., & Lau, K. W. (2017). Effect of aging on stem cells. *World journal of experimental medicine,* 7(1), 1–10. https://doi.org/10.5493/wjem.v7.i1.1

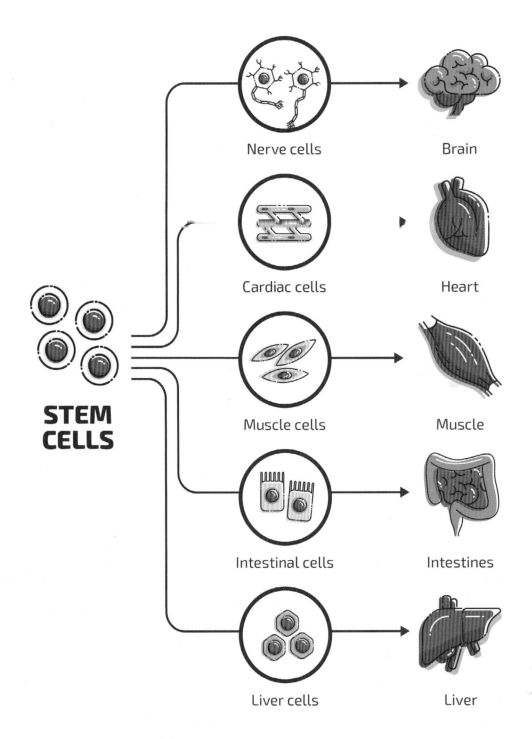

Aging Driver #9: Altered Intercellular Communication

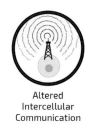

Altered
Intercellular
Communication

Cells communicate between each other back and forth sending signals. Cells operate like an ant colony. Ants send signals to each other by using pheromones, sounds, and touch that allow them to know where to go and other pertinent information.

Imagine an army that loses all communication. It will quickly devolve into chaos. Your body works the same way. For everything to work in harmony, everything from cells to organs needs strong communication capabilities to function properly.

As we age, the signaling environment of chemical messages across the whole body tends to become more inflammatory, inhibiting the immune system and potentially causing muscle wasting, bone loss, and other harmful effects[62] in a process known as inflammaging.

The body is a bio-electro-chemical machine. Many topic-based experts become trapped in either the "biology", "the electricity" or the "chemical" perspectives and biases.

One of the best books written on the body and electricity is called "The Body Electric: Electromagnetism And The Foundation Of Life" by Robert Becker. Most of the communication between our cells, organs, and tissues is facilitated by a signaling process that uses a unique type of electricity.

We believe that one of the keys to improving cellular intercommunication is optimal levels of every macro and micro mineral in the body. It is well known that saltwater is a better conductive fluid than distilled water.

Although yet proven, we also believe that optimal levels of trace minerals are critical to make your cells function at their best and stay strong. We also believe that many of them help with intercellular communication.

Powermove: Optimize Your Mineral Levels

That's why we created Primergen-V and Primergen-M to help supply your cells with all the vitamins and minerals they need to operate at their best.

We strongly recommend consuming a lot of high-quality saltwater (Himalayan or clean sea salt). If you follow a low carb diet, we recommend adding ¼ tsp of cream of tartar with ½ tsp of salt in 2 liters of water and drinking throughout the day. It's easy to become depleted of electrolytes when on a ketogenic diet.

---

62 López-Otín, C., Blasco, M. A., Partridge, L., Serrano, M., & Kroemer, G. (2013). The hallmarks of aging. *Cell*, 153(6), 1194–1217. https://doi.org/10.1016/j.cell.2013.05.039

Of course, consult with your medical experts if you have high blood pressure or other health concerns before starting any new supplement or health protocol.

Aging Driver #10: Enzymatic Depletion

Enzymes do over 25,000 different functions in the human body: everything from thinking to blinking.

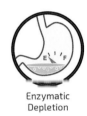

Enzymatic
Depletion

Edwards Howell theorized that humans have an enzyme bank account that gets depleted as we get older. This makes sense when we correlate it to the increase in digestive issues that come with age. Having fewer enzymes and less HCL (stomach acid) all lead to bloating, gas, and other digestive issues.

This leads to a negative cycle of effects. First, this leads to less protein breakdown which means the body gets fewer amino acids. Amino acids are the key building blocks from all the 20,000 proteins and 7,000 peptides your body assembles to make you rock and roll. Eventually, certain functions in the body decline and then cease. Then this creates another negative cascade of events that can lead to serious health issues.

That's why we're such big proponents of enzymes and other digestive aids. They are some of the biggest game-changers anyone can consume to improve their healthspan and lifespan.

The digestive enzymes are only one part of the equation and we will go into great depth on that later in the book.

Powermove: Consume Potent Proteolytic Enzymes

We also believe that consuming lots of proteolytic enzymes on an empty stomach is a powerful anti-aging solution for various reasons.

First, they will break down undigested proteins in your digestive tract and blood. They can start breaking down protein which is accumulating in your cells and disrupting intercellular communication and functions. They can also help reduce inflammation, heal injuries faster, and speed up autophagy.

We believe that MassZymes is the most potent proteolytic enzyme formula on the market.

We live in exciting times. We understand the body at a level we never had before. New breakthroughs in health technology are happening at a record pace. We have more tools at our disposal. We have new ways of testing and optimizing our bodies: DNA, blood tests, sleep monitors, food allergies, gut biome tests, and many more.

Armed with this knowledge, you now have control over your healthspan and can positively impact your lifespan.

We can't make any crazy claims around extending lifespan, however, based on the research and using simple reasoning - we do believe that you can also extend your lifespan by following the information in this book.

By following this blueprint you can:

- Optimize your hormones
- Build and maintain your lean muscle mass
- Increase your drive and motivation
- Improve your sex life
- Maximize the quality of your sleep
- Sharpen your mind and avoid mental decline

It's just a matter of stacking the Powermoves and being consistent. It's that simple.

Chapter 3

Biological Enemy #2: Stress, The Silent Killer

In this chapter, you will learn:

Stress

- **A hidden source of stress that could age you and destroy your happiness.**

- How stress drains your immune system and leaves you vulnerable to attacks.

- **The stress hormone connection: why excess stress shows up around your waistline.**

- And much more...

Stress in the right amount can save lives. Too much stress kills.[63]

Your body's stress response is perfectly normal and critical for your survival. If someone is chasing you with a knife, your body's reaction can be the difference between life or death.

These hormones prepare the body to run away or fight as it draws more oxygen, muscles tighten, the heart beats faster, and breathing accelerates.

The body also suppresses the immune, excretory, and reproductive systems, and it's all to prepare for action. It's obvious that if these critical body functions are compromised long term, dire health consequences will occur.

The Stress Spectrum

Stress response is not a 0 or a 10. It responds in accordance to the perceived threat. The stress response between a bear chasing you in the woods and having a looming deadline at work is not the same. The problem is the majority of people are constantly in a 2-8 range. There is a constant low-to-mid level of stress hormones floating in the body.

---

[63] Society, A. (2020). Stress, *The Silent Killer | American Brain Society.* American Brain Society. Retrieved 2 October 2020, from https://americanbrainsociety.org/stress-the-silent-killer/

The 5 Levels of Stress

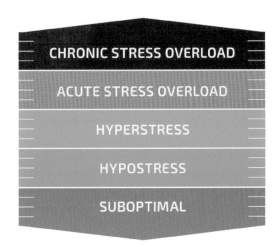

Modern-Day Stress

Almost no one in today's world is being chased by sharks, knives, and tigers. So why is the body having these stress responses?

It's because your brain doesn't differentiate between a physical threat or an emotional threat. The biological response is the same.

When someone loses their job, their mind can start racing and projecting the worst-case scenario. Financial insecurity and fear take hold. Questions like *"What if I can't pay my rent? What if I can't buy food for my family?"* start running through the mind.

When someone leaves a relationship, it's common for the other person to feel insecure. *"What if I'm not good enough? What if I can't attract someone else? What if I'm alone the rest of my life?"*

The core root of these modern stress responses is unprocessed trauma.

When we experience a painful event, unless we "process it" and heal it, it will get stored into the limbic system as a way to protect us in the future. This is how PTSD (post-traumatic stress disorder) happens. The keyword is "traumatic".

How does trauma happen? It usually occurs when 4 conditions are present:

    1 - There's a painful experience.
    2 - It was unexpected.
    3 - The person is unresourced to process it.
    4 - The person feels alone.

When trauma happens, people usually resort to emotional repression and suppression to cope with it. This buries the trauma in the emotional brain and limbic system. Then the amygdala (the security guard of the brain), scans for threats. Any time it sees anything that is remotely close in nature to those old traumas, it will react. The nervous system goes straight to fight, flight, or freeze.

We all know people that have been bitten by a dog and are scared of dogs their entire life. They're 40, 50, or 60 years old and they'll still feel scared of a chihuahua, even if it's friendly. A dog comes into the elevator with them, the adrenal glands get activated. There's sweat, tension goes up, and the heart rate speeds up.

And it's very true even on micro-levels. If your father told you your grades aren't good enough even though you hit 96/100 and he says, *"Where are the other four points?"* Those can be traumatic experiences for a kid. Decades later, when someone even implies that you might NOT be good enough, it can retrigger the same emotional response you had as a kid.

According to experts in the field, it is believed that the average person has between 300 to 500 of these stored traumas in their nervous system. It's no surprise that people are in a constant state of stress and reactivity.

Powermove: EFT and Other Emotional Healing Modalities

Emotional Freedom Techniques (EFT) is a tapping technique based on the 5,000-year-old healing tradition of acupressure for the relief of psychological and physical distress. By tapping on energy points in your body you're able to release blockages and the problem feeling can then be released and move through the body.

In one study, participants experienced significant decreases in anxiety, depression, PTSD, pain, and cravings, and a significant increase in happiness.[64] Another study found similar results, participants showed simultaneous reductions in PTSD, anxiety, and depression symptoms.[65]

EFT is one of the most rapid, economical, and effective ways to process these old buried traumas.

[64] Bach, D., Groesbeck, G., Stapleton, P., Sims, R., Blickheuser, K., & Church, D. (2019). Clinical EFT (Emotional Freedom Techniques) Improves Multiple Physiological Markers of Health. *Journal of evidence-based integrative medicine, 24,* 2515690X18823691. https://doi.org/10.1177/2515690X18823691

[65] Church, D., & House, D. (2018). Borrowing Benefits: Group Treatment With Clinical Emotional Freedom Techniques Is Associated With Simultaneous Reductions in Posttraumatic Stress Disorder, Anxiety, and Depression Symptoms. *Journal of evidence-based integrative medicine,* 23, 2156587218756510. https://doi.org/10.1177/2156587218756510

It's been clinically researched and shown to be extremely effective. It lowers cortisol in minutes. You can learn it in minutes and start applying it in your life immediately.

A great resource to learn more is *www.eftuniverse.com*

Immune System[66]

These traumas can create an immune system and serious health problems.[67] [68] [69]

Here's what Emily Deans MD states, *"(Research has shown that) higher lifetime trauma was associated with higher levels of inflammatory cytokines at baseline and 5 years later. When the researchers controlled for psychological symptoms of the trauma (for example, PTSD or clinical depression), the relationship held, meaning those who had undergone trauma had elevations of inflammation even if their behavior and coping seemed more normal by psychiatric diagnostic standards. In these folks with pre-existing cardiovascular disease, higher inflammation is associated with greater risk of death and complication."*

The Goal: Cycling Through Stress

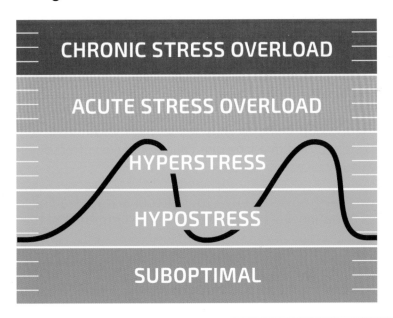

66 Stanford University Medical Center. (2012, June 21). How stress can boost immune system. *ScienceDaily*. Retrieved October 1, 2020 from www.sciencedaily.com/releases/2012/06/120621223525.htm

67 *Stress: The Killer Disease*. Psychology Today. (2020). Retrieved 2 October 2020, from https://www.psychologytoday.com/us/blog/evolutionary-psychiatry/201211/stress-the-killer-disease.

68 George, A. (2020). *Cytokine storm*. New Scientist. Retrieved 2 October 2020, from https://www.newscientist.com/term/cytokine-storm/.

69 *Stress: The Killer Disease*. Psychology Today. (2020). Retrieved 2 October 2020, from https://www.psychologytoday.com/us/blog/evolutionary-psychiatry/201211/stress-the-killer-disease.

The goal is to spend most of your time at low levels of stress and then increase it when needed for special occasions. Getting amped up for an epic workout is great. Staying stressed every waking hour will destroy your life, short-term and long-term.

The goal isn't to live a stress-free life. The goal is to pay attention to your mind and body and give it what it needs. Your body needs positive stressors (hormetic stress) in order to be as strong and healthy as possible. Your mind needs challenges in order for it to stay sharp.

However, we are not cyborgs. The human mind and body has limits and when we approach those limits, it's wise to pull the stress back and focus on recovery and rejuvenation.

As you can see in the diagram above, you want to cycle through hypostress (low levels of stress) to hyperstress (high manageable levels of stress). When your mind and body hit acute stress overload BACK OFF… And when your stress becomes too low and you feel laziness start to creep in, it's time to start ramping up physical and mental challenges.

Here are some of the consequences of chronic stress.

Blood Sugar Problems

Under stress, your liver produces more blood sugar to give you a boost of energy. If your blood sugar levels are chronically elevated it may increase your risk of developing type 2 diabetes. It can make it very difficult to lose weight in this condition. We will cover various methods of managing your blood sugar in chapter 10.

Digestive Problems

When your body is stressed, blood shifts to muscles to help you mobilize. This can lead to digestive problems. Stress doesn't cause ulcers (a bacterium called H. pylori often does), but it can increase your risk for them and cause existing ulcers to act up.

Stress can also affect the way food moves through your intestinal tract, leading to diarrhea or constipation. We will cover various ways of optimizing your digestion in the latter half of the book.

Powermove: Mindful Eating

Mindful eating can reduce stress and optimize digestion.[70]

This is maintaining an in-the-moment awareness of the food and drink you're consuming. Focus on how the food makes you feel and the signals your body sends about taste, satisfaction, and fullness.

Vascular Health Problems

Stress hormones affect your respiratory and cardiovascular systems. Under stress, your heart pumps faster and stress hormones cause your blood vessels to constrict, which leads to higher blood pressure. When your blood pressure rises, so do your risks of having a stroke or heart attack.[71]

Your muscles tense up in preparation for fight or flight when you're stressed. If you're constantly under stress, your muscles may not get the chance to relax. This can lead to knots and biomechanical dysfunctions. When neck and back muscles tighten up, it can lead to structural problems. Your body can start compensating and your spine, shoulders, and neck can go out of alignment.[72]

Powermove: Get Regular Bodywork

Exercise is essential for better overall health and is also effective in reducing stress.[73] It's important to pick an activity you enjoy so you can stick with it.

Just as important as exercise is recovery. During recovery is when the most muscle is built, because muscle protein synthesis increases by 50% four hours after a workout (like resistance training).[74]

[70] Cherpak C. E. (2019). Mindful Eating: A Review Of How The Stress-Digestion-Mindfulness Triad May Modulate And Improve Gastrointestinal And Digestive Function. *Integrative medicine (Encinitas, Calif.),* 18(4), 48–53.

[71] *The Effects of Stress on Your Body.* Healthline. Retrieved 2 October 2020, from https://www.healthline.com/health/stress/effects-on-body#1.

[72] *Stress Effects on the Body: Musculoskeletal.* https://www.apa.org. Retrieved 2 October 2020, from https://www.apa.org/help-center/stress/effects-musculoskeletal.

[73] Edenfield, T. M., & Blumenthal, J. A. (2011). Exercise and stress reduction. In R. J. Contrada & A. Baum (Eds.), The handbook of stress science: Biology, psychology, and health (p. 301–319). Springer Publishing Company.

[74] Elliot, T. A., Cree, M. G., Sanford, A. P., Wolfe, R. R., & Tipton, K. D. (2006). Milk ingestion stimulates net muscle protein synthesis following resistance exercise. *Medicine and science in sports and exercise,* 38(4), 667–674. https://doi.org/10.1249/01.mss.0000210190.64458.25

> Regular physical activity will provide other gains including weight control and reduced risk of heart disease.

Brain Related Stress Problems

Stress can kill brain cells and even reduce the size of the brain. Cortisol has a shrinking effect on the prefrontal cortex, the area of the brain responsible for memory and learning.[75]

Chronic stress can blow out your hippocampus and wipe out your short-term memory. It may even reduce the size of the hippocampus.

Brain Damage

These changes can lead to decreased spatial and verbal memory abilities. These negative changes in the amygdala and hippocampus can result in decreased decision-making and processing abilities and difficulty learning.[76] **In other words, stress makes you DUMBER.**

Extra Body Fat

Multiple studies confirm a direct correlation between stress and weight gain.[77] When you're stressed, your adrenal glands secrete cortisol, leading to higher levels of this hormone in the body. The cortisol release affects fat distribution by causing fat to be stored centrally-around the organs such as intestines, liver, and kidneys increasing visceral fat.[78]

One study found that stress causes excess abdominal fat in slender women.[79] Another study of stressed-out middle-aged Swedish men similarly showed that those with the highest cortisol levels also had the

[75] Bernstein, R. (2016). *The Mind and Mental Health: How Stress Affects the Brain.* Touro University WorldWide. Retrieved 2 October 2020, from https://www.tuw.edu/health/how-stress-affects-the-brain/.
[76] Smith, S. How EFT Intervenes in Chronic Stress. EFT Universe Learn EFT Tapping Emotional Freedom Techniques. Retrieved 2 October 2020, from https://www.eftuniverse.com/anxiety-stress/how-eft-intervenes-in-chronic-stress.
[77] Jackson, S. E., Kirschbaum, C., & Steptoe, A. (2017). Hair cortisol and adiposity in a population-based sample of 2,527 men and women aged 54 to 87 years. *Obesity (Silver Spring, Md.),* 25(3), 539–544. https://doi.org/10.1002/oby.21733
[78] Goldstein D. S. (2010). Adrenal responses to stress. *Cellular and molecular neurobiology,* 30(8), 1433–1440. https://doi.org/10.1007/s10571-010-9606-9
[79] Epel, E. S., McEwen, B., Seeman, T., Matthews, K., Castellazzo, G., Brownell, K. D., Bell, J., & Ickovics, J. R. (2000). Stress and body shape: stress-induced cortisol secretion is consistently greater among women with central fat. *Psychosomatic medicine,* 62(5), 623–632. https://doi.org/10.1097/00006842-200009000-00005

biggest beer bellies.[80] Furthermore, cortisol has been found to slow down your metabolism, making it difficult to lose weight. The researchers found that, on average, women who reported one or more stressors during the prior 24 hours burned 104 fewer calories than non-stressed women.[81]

Powermove: Meditation

Mindful meditation is an effective treatment for a variety of psychological problems and is especially effective for reducing anxiety, depression, and stress.[82]

The Solutions Are Simple

The solutions to this biological enemy are simple. They are throughout this book. The solution chapters on lean muscle mass, sleep, movement, nervous system optimization, and brain optimization will solve your stress challenges. Pay special attention to the chapter on nervous system optimization because that is the most direct way to manage stress properly.

Conclusion

An acute short-term stress response is ok. The health problems begin when these stress compounds are chronically elevated.

80 Rosmond, R., & Björntorp, P. (2000). Occupational status, cortisol secretory pattern, and visceral obesity in middle-aged men. *Obesity research,* 8(6), 445–450. https://doi.org/10.1038/oby.2000.55
81 Kiecolt-Glaser, J. K., Habash, D. L., Fagundes, C. P., Andridge, R., Peng, J., Malarkey, W. B., & Belury, M. A. (2015). Daily stressors, past depression, and metabolic responses to high-fat meals: a novel path to obesity. *Biological psychiatry,* 77(7), 653–660. https://doi.org/10.1016/j.biopsych.2014.05.018
82 Khoury, B., Lecomte, T., Fortin, G., Masse, M., Therien, P., Bouchard, V., Chapleau, M. A., Paquin, K., & Hofmann, S. G. (2013). Mindfulness-based therapy: a comprehensive meta-analysis. *Clinical psychology review,* 33(6), 763–771. https://doi.org/10.1016/j.cpr.2013.05.005

Chapter 4

Biological Enemy #3: Toxins

In this chapter, you will learn:

- **Why toxins play a role in nearly every chronic health condition.**

- Little-known sources of toxins that "sneak" their way into healthy lifestyles.

- **How to detoxify and remove pollutants on a deep cellular level without harsh cleanses.**

- And much more...

Deficiency

We hear a lot of information in the news today about toxins. Whether it's heavy metals, pollutants from the air, food additives, preservatives, or genetically modified foods.

We define a toxin as anything that interrupts the optimal metabolic functions of the body. If toxins reach certain levels in our bodies, they become lethal. This is why it's important to minimize them from our environments and eliminate them from our bodies.

In the case of athletic excellence, fitness, or health optimization, toxins inhibit your ability to perform at its highest capabilities. Most of us have been hungover from a party. We weren't going to win any Gold Medals that day.

Let's use an example of a common toxin that virtually everybody's exposed to, chlorine. Chlorine has been used to kill bacteria in water and it's been very successful. But after 30 or 40 years of using chlorine, scientists discovered that it's correlated with cancer rates.[83]

Powermove: Use Powerful Whole House Water Filters

We suggest buying powerful water filters that remove the majority of the key toxins that are found in water. Do your research and choose a filter that removes chlorine and fluoride.

If you put chlorine next to a bacteria culture, it kills bacteria. So if I'm drinking chlorinated water, that chlorine is now going into my digestive tract and wiping out good AND bad bacteria. It's not differentiating between the two.

---

[83] Morris RD. Drinking water and cancer. Environ Health Perspect. 1995 Nov;103 Suppl 8(Suppl 8):225-31. doi: 10.1289/ehp.95103s8225. PMID: 8741788; PMCID: PMC1518976.

Our intestinal flora (good bacteria) is essential for digesting and assimilating food, as well as defending you against viruses and toxic bacteria.

Fluoride is another example. It's present in 99% of toothpastes and can block "T4-T3 hormone conversion", which is critical for healthy thyroid function.[84]

Powermove: Use Fluoride-Free Toothpastes

We suggest using fluoride-free toothpaste and other toxin-free skincare, shampoos, and chemical-free cosmetics. The majority of popular toothpastes have fluoride and other known toxic additives.

Additionally, here are some other toxins most people don't think about on a regular basis:

- Mercury from amalgam fillings, which a lot of people have, can compromise brain chemistry,[85] and may cause unnatural cell mutation and brain damage.[86]

- Prescription drugs like antibiotics don't discriminate between good bacteria and bad bacteria. They're wiping out the good with the bad, which has an impact on our digestive health and immunity.

Any time you destroy your intestinal flora with antibiotics, two things happen:

1 - Your digestion is impaired. Your body will struggle to break down and absorb the nutrients from your food.

2 - Your body loses its primary defenders. Your body becomes vulnerable against viruses, bad bacteria, and other invaders. In this state, it's easy for your body to catch the flu and get sick.

Another serious potential problem that has been proven to occur with various toxins is bacterial mutation.

For instance, It was recently discovered that one of the reasons artificial sweeteners can create health

[84] GE, Y., NING, H., GU, X., YIN, M., YANG, X., QI, Y., & WANG, J. (2013). Effects of High Fluoride and Low Iodine on Thyroid Function in Offspring Rats. *Journal Of Integrative Agriculture,* 12(3), 502-508. https://doi.org/10.1016/s2095-3119(13)60251-8
[85] Fernandes Azevedo, B., Barros Furieri, L., Peçanha, F. M., Wiggers, G. A., Frizera Vassallo, P., Ronacher Simões, M., Fiorim, J., Rossi de Batista, P., Fioresi, M., Rossoni, L., Stefanon, I., Alonso, M. J., Salaices, M., & Valentim Vassallo, D. (2012). Toxic effects of mercury on the cardiovascular and central nervous systems. *Journal of biomedicine & biotechnology,* 2012, 949048. https://doi.org/10.1155/2012/949048
[86] Huggins, H., & Levy, T. (1999). *Uninformed consent.* Hampton Roads Pub. Co.

problems is because the intestinal flora becomes glucose resistant within 1 week of daily artificial sweetener consumption.[87]

In another study, it was shown that GMO (genetically modified) food created a mutation of the bacteria.[88]

What are the long term consequences of these gut biome mutations? No one's certain - but it's probably not good.

An Eye-Opening Look at the Toxins in Our Lives

Here's a brief look at what we're up against when it comes to toxins impairing our attainment of biological optimization.

25 Sources Of Toxins Found in Food, Pharmaceuticals, and Life

Here are brief summaries of 25 studies that reveal just a small sample of the toxicities we're facing today along with 25 Powermoves to help you deal with them.

1 - Heavy metals in plants you consume have an impact on your health.

"Dietary intake of many heavy metals through consumption of plants has long term detrimental effects on human health." [89]

Heavy metals are present in nature. Therefore, they accumulate in soils and plants interfering with the levels of antioxidants in plants and reducing the nutritive value of the produce.

Certain crops such as spinach, lettuce, carrot, radish, and zucchini can accumulate heavy metals in their tissues.[90] This means the metals cannot be removed by washing or rinsing.

[87] Suez, J., Korem, T., Zeevi, D., Zilberman-Schapira, G., Thaiss, C. A., Maza, O., Israeli, D., Zmora, N., Gilad, S., Weinberger, A., Kuperman, Y., Harmelin, A., Kolodkin-Gal, I., Shapiro, H., Halpern, Z., Segal, E., & Elinav, E. (2014). Artificial sweeteners induce glucose intolerance by altering the gut microbiota. *Nature, 514*(7521), 181–186. https://doi.org/10.1038/nature13793
[88] Kleter, G. A., Peijnenburg, A. A., & Aarts, H. J. (2005). Health considerations regarding horizontal transfer of microbial transgenes present in genetically modified crops. *Journal of biomedicine & biotechnology*, 2005(4), 326–352. https://doi.org/10.1155/JBB.2005.326
[89] Sharma, R. K., & Agrawal, M. (2005). Biological effects of heavy metals: an overview. *Journal of environmental biology*, 26(2 Suppl), 301–313.
[90] Intawongse, M., & Dean, J. R. (2006). Uptake of heavy metals by vegetable plants grown on contaminated soil and their bioavailability in the human gastrointestinal tract. *Food additives and contaminants*, 23(1), 36–48. https://doi.org/10.1080/02652030500387554

Powermove: Sweat

Saunas and sweating are great ways of removing heavy metals out of the body. Other products that have shown to be effective include Cytodetox and Biosil.

2 - Pesticides may have cancer-causing potential.

"The most significant harmful effects come from fertilizer that is designed to kill or prevent weeds. According to the EPA's Office of Pesticide Programs, 12 of the most popular pesticides in the United States have ingredients known to cause cancer." [91]

Powermove: Eat Organic

Organic foods have more nutrients and antioxidants than conventionally-grown produce. More importantly, you'll avoid a host of chemicals that we frankly don't know what the real consequences are.

If you can't afford organic foods, we suggest avoiding the dirty dozen, which are 12 crops that farmers use the most pesticides on:

Strawberries, spinach, nectarines, apples, grapes, peaches, cherries, pears, tomatoes, celery, potatoes, and sweet bell peppers.

3 - Pollutants in the soil spread throughout the food chain.

"Soil that is not significantly polluted may still harm humans indirectly, according to Pollution Issues. One way such soil pollution can harm humans is by bioaccumulation. Plants that are grown in lightly polluted soil continuously absorb molecules of the pollutants. Since the plants cannot get rid of these molecules, they accumulate in the plant, causing higher amounts of pollution to exist in the plant than in the soil. Animals who eat many of these polluted plants take on all the pollution those plants have accumulated. Larger animals who eat the plant-eating animals take on all the pollution from the animals they eat. Humans who eat plants or

---

[91] Aktar, M. W., Sengupta, D., & Chowdhury, A. (2009). Impact of pesticides use in agriculture: their benefits and hazards. *Interdisciplinary toxicology,* 2(1), 1–12. https://doi.org/10.2478/v10102-009-0001-7

animals that have accumulated large amounts of soil pollutants may be poisoned, even if the soil itself does not contain enough pollution to harm human health." [92]

Powermove: Dry Skin Brushing to Detox

Dry brushing stimulates the lymphatic system to remove cell waste, environmental toxins, and pathogenic organisms more efficiently.[93] It is recommended to take a natural, soft-bristled brush and start from the extremities (feet and hands) and move toward the center of the body as you brush. Do this before your shower or sauna and then wash off the dead skin after.

4 - Sugar intake may depress immune response.

"Excess sugar depresses immunity. Studies have shown that downing 75 to 100 grams of a sugar solution (about 20 teaspoons of sugar, or the amount that is contained in two average 12-ounce sodas or 2 legendary Cronuts™) can suppress the body's immune responses. Simple sugars, including glucose, table sugar, fructose, and honey caused a fifty- percent drop in the ability of white blood cells to engulf bacteria." [94]

Powermove: Power Walk After a Sweet Indulgence

A quick 10 min walk, especially after you have any meal that is rich in carbohydrates or anything with sugar (natural or otherwise), will do wonders for your blood sugar. More on that in chapter 10.

5 - Brain development and behavior may be impacted by antibiotics given to food animals.

"There is an increasing amount of evidence suggesting that the sub-therapeutic use of antibiotics in food

92 *Soil Pollution.* Everything Connects. (2013). Retrieved 2 October 2020, from https://www.everythingconnects.org/soil-pollution.html.

93 *Dry Brushing: Benefits, Risks, and More.* Healthline. (2017). Retrieved 2 October 2020, from https://www.healthline.com/health/dry-brushing.

94 Sears, D. *Harmful Effects of Excess Sugar.* Ask Dr Sears. Retrieved 2 October 2020, from https://www.askdrsears.com/topics/feeding-eating/family-nutrition/sugar/harmful-effects-excess-sugar.

animals can pose a health risk to humans. If a group of animals is treated with a certain antibiotic over time, the bacteria living in those animals will become resistant to that drug. According to microbiologist Dr. Glenn Morris, the problem for humans is that if a person ingests the resistant bacteria, they have a significant impact on brain development and subsequent adult behavior." [95]

Powermove: Load up on Probiotics When Doing Antibiotics

If you do antibiotics, it is extra beneficial to consume probiotics before, during, and after the course of antibiotics to replenish healthy gut flora levels. Based on our lab test, the probiotics inside of Biome Breakthrough have been shown to be resistant to antibiotics which makes it a good option when doing antibiotics.

6 - Artificial sweeteners may disrupt blood sugar regulation.

"Artificial sweeteners may disrupt the body's ability to regulate blood sugar, causing metabolic changes that can be a precursor to diabetes, researchers are reporting." [96]

Powermove: Consume Natural Sweeteners

There are some really tasty natural sweeteners including erythritol, monk fruit, allulose, and stevia. We live in a time of unparalleled options when it comes to healthy, natural alternatives. Most health food stores have dozens of choices that can replace virtually any product with tasty sweeteners. If you're craving sodas, we recommend either Zevia or other flavored waters like LaCroix.

[95] Landers, T. F., Cohen, B., Wittum, T. E., & Larson, E. L. (2012). A review of antibiotic use in food animals: perspective, policy, and potential. *Public health reports (Washington, D.C. : 1974), 127*(1), 4–22. https://doi.org/10.1177/003335491212700103

[96] Suez, J., Korem, T., Zeevi, D., Zilberman-Schapira, G., Thaiss, C. A., Maza, O., Israeli, D., Zmora, N., Gilad, S., Weinberger, A., Kuperman, Y., Harmelin, A., Kolodkin-Gal, I., Shapiro, H., Halpern, Z., Segal, E., & Elinav, E. (2014). Artificial sweeteners induce glucose intolerance by altering the gut microbiota. *Nature, 514*(7521), 181–186. https://doi.org/10.1038/nature13793

7 - Over 3,000 preservatives, flavorings, colors, and food ingredients do not require testing for estrogenic activity.

"More than 3,000 preservatives, flavorings, colors, and other ingredients are added to food in the United States, and none of them are required to undergo testing for estrogenic activity, according to the Food and Drug Administration."

"We need to be mindful of these food additives because they could be adding to the total effect of other estrogen-mimicking compounds we're coming into contact with," said Clair Hicks, a professor of food science at the University of Kentucky and spokesperson for the Institute of Food Technologists, a nonprofit scientific group. [97]

Powermove: Use Glass

Glass jars contain no chemicals, therefore can be safely washed at high temperatures without harmful chemicals leaching into food, unlike plastic. Use glass or metal containers for your water. There's no reason to use plastics to store anything.

8 - Genetically engineered foods may lead to leaky gut syndrome.

"Genetically engineered food genes transferring to the bacteria in our guts could lead to problems like leaky gut syndrome: Leaky gut syndrome happens when the intestinal lining becomes inflamed, and the microvilli on the lining become damaged; this prevents the microvilli from absorbing nutrients and producing necessary enzymes and secretions for healthy digestion and absorption." [98]

Powermove: Use Biome Breakthrough

Biome Breakthrough® is an incredibly powerful formula that can repair and rebuild compromised gut-lining. We've proven in our lab that it's extremely effective at building biofilm.

---

[97] Amadasi, A., Mozzarelli, A., Meda, C., Maggi, A., & Cozzini, P. (2009). Identification of xenoestrogens in food additives by an integrated in silico and in vitro approach. *Chemical research in toxicology,* 22(1), 52–63. https://doi.org/10.1021/tx800048m

[98] *Genetically Engineered Food Alters Our Digestive Systems.* The Alliance for Natural Health. (2011). Retrieved 2 October 2020, from https://anh-usa.org/genetically-engineered-food-alters-our-digestive-systems/.

9 - Gluten may be linked with neurological disorders.

"The main neurological disorder believed to be at least partly caused by gluten is cerebellar ataxia, a serious disease of the brain that involves an inability to coordinate balance, movements, problems talking. It is now known that many cases of ataxia are directly linked to gluten consumption. This... gluten ataxia involves irreversible damage to the cerebellum, a part of the brain that is important in motor control." [99]

Powermove: Avoid or Minimize Gluten

However, if you're unable to steer clear of gluten (most often when dining out or traveling), take Gluten Guardian with the meal and then take Biome Breakthrough the next day.

Gluten Guardian is a blend of plant-based proteolytic enzymes that break down starches and sugars. Biome Breakthrough combines the right probiotics and prebiotics for optimal gut health, reduces gut inflammation, and eliminates bloating and gas.

10 - Artificial food coloring may have an impact on behavior.

The link between artificial colors and behavioral problems is a concern, especially for parents of children diagnosed with ADHD. The safety of products containing artificial colors has been a point of debate for decades – adversaries claiming that they are toxic, carcinogens, and contributors to ADHD. [100]

Powermove: Avoid Artificial Color Additives

Who knows what these are doing to us? When purchasing a product, read the label to make sure it does not include artificial colors. The most common are Blue No. 1, Yellow No. 5, and Yellow No. 6.

There are now many snack foods that don't use dye coloring, which makes for a much healthier option.

99 Hadjivassiliou, M., Sanders, D. S., Woodroofe, N., Williamson, C., & Grünewald, R. A. (2008). Gluten ataxia. *Cerebellum (London, England)*, 7(3), 494–498. https://doi.org/10.1007/s12311-008-0052-x
100 Arnold, L. E., Lofthouse, N., & Hurt, E. (2012). Artificial food colors and attention-deficit/hyperactivity symptoms: conclusions to dye for. *Neurotherapeutics : the journal of the American Society for Experimental NeuroTherapeutics*, 9(3), 599–609. https://doi.org/10.1007/s13311-012-0133-x

11 - Synthetic vitamin behavior may be different from natural vitamins.

Even though the chemistry may be identical there is a significant difference between man-made and natural nutrition. Light passing through a natural vitamin always bends to the right due to its molecular rotation. This is a (d) configuration for dextrorotatory. Synthetic vitamins behave differently. [101]

Powermove:
Try to Get Your Vitamins from Food as Much as Possible

If you're going to take a nutritional supplement, it must be high quality such as Primergen-M and Primergen-V that combine fulvic acid for up to 98% absorption.

12 - Slaughterhouse meat is contaminated with E.Coli bacteria.

A very high percentage of all the flesh from animals butchered every year in the U.S. is contaminated with E.coli, campylobacter, listeria, or other dangerous bacteria that live in the intestinal tracts, flesh, and feces of animals.[102]

Every year in the U.S., there are 75 million cases of food poisoning, and 5,000 of these cases are fatal. The U.S. Department of Agriculture (USDA) reports that 70 percent of food poisoning is caused by contaminated animal flesh.[103]

Powermove: Eat Grass-Fed/Wild Meat

Grass-fed meat is meat that comes from cows or livestock that eat grass (their natural diet) rather than grains. The result is a much more favorable ratio of nutrients and essential fatty acids (including omega-3s and CLA) than in animals that have been fed an unnatural grain diet.

[101] Jockers, D. (2011). *Understand the difference between synthetic and whole food supplementation.* Drhansenchiropractic.com. Retrieved 2 October 2020, from https://www.drhansenchiropractic.com/blog/9023-understand-the-difference-between-synthetic-and-whole-food-supplementation.

[102] Gansheroff, L. J., & O'Brien, A. D. (2000). Escherichia coli O157:H7 in beef cattle presented for slaughter in the U.S.: higher prevalence rates than previously estimated. *Proceedings of the National Academy of Sciences of the United States of America, 97*(7), 2959–2961. https://doi.org/10.1073/pnas.97.7.2959

[103] Hedberg C. (1999). Food-related illness and death in the United States. *Emerging infectious diseases, 5*(6), 840–842. https://doi.org/10.3201/eid0506.990624

13 - Prevalence of fecal matter in ground beef.

"A nationwide study published by the USDA in 1996 found that 78.6 percent of the ground beef contained microbes that are spread primarily by fecal matter. The medical literature on the causes of food poisoning is full of euphemisms and dry scientific terms: coliform levels, aerobic plate counts, sorbitol, MacConkey agar, and so on. Behind them lies a simple explanation for why eating hamburger meat makes you sick: There is shit in the meat.") [106]

Powermove: Consume P3-OM With Each Meal

P3OM has been shown to defeat bacteria that cause food poisoning including e.coli.

It's a great supplement to take when you're not sure the food is clean and when you're traveling.

14 - Soy supplementation and cancer risk.

94 percent of soybeans are genetically engineered in the US, according to the Center for Food Safety, which makes it the number one GM crop plant in the world.

The problem with this is, almost all genetically modified soybeans are designed to be "Roundup ready" - they're engineered to withstand heavy doses of herbicides that kill any unwanted vegetation but not the soybean plant itself. The main active ingredient in Roundup, glyphosate has been labeled as probably carcinogenic to humans.

Researchers found that genetically engineered soybeans accumulate and absorb high levels of glyphosate, which cannot be removed by rinsing.[107] Studies in animals using human cells have found serious negative health effects at concentrations far below the MRLs (maximum residue level), including causing miscarriages and abnormal fetal development by interfering with hormone productions.[108]

[106] Schlosser, E., & Wilson, C. (2006). *Chew on this.* Penguin.
[107] Bøhn, T., Cuhra, M., Traavik, T., Sanden, M., Fagan, J., & Primicerio, R. (2014). Compositional differences in soybeans on the market: glyphosate accumulates in Roundup Ready GM soybeans. *Food chemistry, 153,* 207–215. https://doi.org/10.1016/j.foodchem.2013.12.054
[108] de Araujo, J. S., Delgado, I. F., & Paumgartten, F. J. (2016). Glyphosate and adverse pregnancy outcomes, a systematic review of observational studies. *BMC public health, 16,* 472. https://doi.org/10.1186/s12889-016-3153-3

Powermove: Avoid or Minimize Soy

We suggest avoiding or minimizing soy supplements, soy-based foods, soy protein, and soy-fed animals until more research is done.[109] The only exception would be fermented, probiotic-rich soy foods like tamari, miso, natto, and others.

15 - Mercury found in fish and shellfish are a bigger concern than many believe.

Mercury found in fish and shellfish is considered by WHO as one of the top ten chemicals or groups of chemicals of major public health concern. [110]

Canned white albacore tuna typically has higher levels of mercury than canned light tuna.

Studies show that high exposure to mercury induces changes in the central nervous system, potentially resulting in irritability, fatigue, behavioral changes, tremors, headaches, hearing and cognitive loss, dysarthria, incoordination, hallucinations, and death.[111]

Powermove: Avoid Farm Fish as Much as Possible

If you're going to eat sushi, choose wild salmon. King mackerel, marlin, orange roughy, shark, swordfish, tilefish, ahi tuna, and bigeye tuna all contain high levels of mercury.

Doing frequent sauna sessions have also been shown to be effective at reducing heavy metals in the body.

---

[109] *Soy and Cancer Risk: Our Expert's Advice.* Cancer.org. (2012). Retrieved 2 October 2020, from https://www.cancer.org/lat-est-news/soy-and-cancer-risk-our-experts-advice.html.
[110] *Mercury and health.* Who.int. (2017). Retrieved 2 October 2020, from https://www.who.int/news-room/fact-sheets/detail/mercury-and-health#:~:text=Mercury%20is%20considered%20by%20WHO,shellfish%20that%20contain%20the%20compound.
[111] Fernandes Azevedo, B., Barros Furieri, L., Peçanha, F. M., Wiggers, G. A., Frizera Vassallo, P., Ronacher Simões, M., Fiorim, J., Rossi de Batista, P., Fioresi, M., Rossoni, L., Stefanon, I., Alonso, M. J., Salaices, M., & Valentim Vassallo, D. (2012). Toxic effects of mercury on the cardiovascular and central nervous systems. *Journal of biomedicine & biotechnology, 2012,* 949048. https://doi.org/10.1155/2012/949048

16 - Our drinking water can be contaminated from a number of sources.

"Dirty water is the world's biggest health risk and continues to threaten both quality of life and public health in the United States. When water from rain and melting snow runs off roofs and roads into our rivers, it picks up toxic chemicals, dirt, trash, and disease-carrying organisms along the way. Many of our water resources also lack basic protections, making them vulnerable to pollution from factory farms, industrial plants, and activities like fracking." [112]

If you haven't watched the movie "Dark Waters" or seen the Netflix documentary "The Devil We Know", we strongly suggest you do. It's shocking and eye opening.

Powermove: Filter Your Water

Add multiple water filters to your house water systems.
We suggest adding whole house filters as well as water optimizers for your tap.

17 - Vitamin D deficiency may be linked to sunscreen use.

"According to the CDC, in 2006 a whopping one-fourth of the population was deficient in vitamin D. Eight percent were "at-risk" for vitamin D deficiency illnesses and one percent had levels that were considered imminently harmful. [113]

What's causing this epidemic of low vitamin D levels? One theory is that we are not outside as much as prior generations, and when we are, we slather on the sunscreen which prohibits UVB (the rays responsible for suntans) from penetrating the skin. These same UVB rays naturally produce vitamin D." [114]

Powermove: Get in the Sun

We strongly recommend getting 15-20 minutes of sun every day without sunscreen.
See Chapter 16 for more insights.

[112] *Water Pollution.* NRDC. Retrieved 2 October 2020, from https://www.nrdc.org/issues/water-pollution.
[113] Looker, A. C., Johnson, C. L., Lacher, D. A., Pfeiffer, C. M., Schleicher, R. L., & Sempos, C. T. (2011). Vitamin D status: United States, 2001-2006. *NCHS data brief,* (59), 1–8.
[114] *Vitamin D Deficiency and Depression.* Psychology Today. (2013). Retrieved 2 October 2020, from https://www.psychologyto-day.com/ca/blog/reading-between-the-headlines/201307/vitamin-d-deficiency-and-depression?ampdepression=.

18 - Dangerous chemicals lurk in makeup beauty products.

"Since 2009, 604 cosmetics manufacturers have reported using 95 chemicals, in more than 85,515 products, that have been linked to cancer, birth defects or reproductive harm." [115]

Powermove: Use Chemical-Free Cosmetics

Go to *ewg.org* to look up the products you use and find out if they're safe. You can also search for low toxin options.

19 - There are reports of neurological effects resulting from mercury in dental routines.

"Dr. Hal Huggins, an expert dentist in mercury removal, reports on numerous psychological disorders that appear to be the effect of mercury in amalgams, including but not limited to, borderline personality disorder, depression, anxiety, insanity of all kinds, schizophrenia, panic attacks and obsessive-compulsive disorder (OCD)." [116]

Powermove: Get Your Mercury Fillings Replaced

If you have mercury amalgams, get your mercury replaced by a natural or biological dentist. Ceramic or zirconium fillings contain no metals and are generally much healthier options compared to mercury fillings.

20 - The overuse of antibiotics is resulting in the occurrence of "superbugs".

"Infections we thought we had conquered once and for all are coming back because of a new breed of germs that doctors call "superbugs" -- bacteria that are resistant to almost all antibiotics. The latest culprit is called MRSA, a staph bacteria that triggers infections so virulent they can - and have - turned deadly within days." [117]

[115] Bergfeld, W. F., Belsito, D. V., Marks, J. G., Jr, & Andersen, F. A. (2005). Safety of ingredients used in cosmetics. *Journal of the American Academy of Dermatology, 52*(1), 125–132. https://doi.org/10.1016/j.jaad.2004.07.066

[116] Huggins, H. (1993). *It's all in your head.* Avery Pub. Group.

[117] *Super-Resistant Superbugs.* Cbsnews.com. (2004). Retrieved 2 October 2020, from https://www.cbsnews.com/news/super-resistant-superbugs/.

Powermove: Keep Your Immune System Strong

The best answer against many pathogens is a strong immune system. Following the suggestions in this book will help you maximize your immune strength. Biome Breakthrough also helps provide a powerful immune boost.

21 - Pharmaceutical drugs are toxic.

Many drugs create unwanted side-effects: illnesses, toxicity, and death. [118]

"Deaths from drug overdose have been rising steadily over the past two decades and have become the leading cause of injury death in the United States." [119]

Powermove: Start With Natural Solutions

We live in a time where natural solutions have become incredibly concentrated and powerful. For almost every health issue, there is usually a natural solution, supplement, or other modality that can solve your health challenge without needing pharmaceuticals. Of course, consult with your health practitioner.

22 - Our respiratory health can be impacted by our living spaces.

"There is mounting evidence that exposure to IAQ (indoor air quality) is the cause of excessive morbidity and mortality. In the developed world IAQ is a main cause of allergies, other hypersensitivity reactions, airway infections, and cancers." [120]

[118] Seagrave, Z., & Bamba, S. (2017). Adverse drug reactions. *Disease-a-month : DM, 63*(2), 49–53. https://doi.org/10.1016/j.disamonth.2016.09.006

[119] *Poisoning. Home and Recreational Safety.* CDC Injury Center. Cdc.gov. (2015). Retrieved 2 October 2020, from https://www.cdc.gov/homeandrecreationalsafety/poisoning/index.html.

[120] Sundell J. (2004). On the history of indoor air quality and health. *Indoor air, 14 Suppl 7,* 51–58. https://doi.org/10.1111/j.1600-0668.2004.00273.x

Powermove: Get Air Filters

We suggest using air filters in your bedroom, office, or any other room you spend a lot of time in. There are plenty of high-quality HEPA air filters that are effective.

23 - Obesogens contribute to obesity.

Obesogens are chemicals that may disrupt our bodies' naturally occurring metabolic processes and may predispose someone to gain weight. Obesogens can be found in most common household products, cosmetics, plastics, pesticides, our food supply and water supply.

"Obesogens have been linked to obesity birth defects, premature puberty in girls, demasculinization in men, breast cancer and other disorders." [121]

Powermove: Reduce Your Exposure to Obesogens

As stated in earlier Powermoves, steer clear of chemical-laded cosmetics, water, foods and beverages.

24 - EMF radiation is detrimental to our overall health.

"EMF radiation affects sleep quality because it reduces the amount of melatonin we produce." [122]

Chronic sleep deprivation can have serious potential health problems, including increased risk for stroke, obesity, diabetes, cancer, permanent cognitive deficits, osteoporosis, cardiovascular disease, and mortality. [123]

[121] Darbre P. D. (2017). Endocrine Disruptors and Obesity. *Current obesity reports, 6*(1), 18–27. https://doi.org/10.1007/s13679-017-0240-4

[122] Halgamuge M. N. (2013). Pineal melatonin level disruption in humans due to electromagnetic fields and ICNIRP limits. *Radiation protection dosimetry, 154*(4), 405–416. https://doi.org/10.1093/rpd/ncs255

[123] Abrams R. M. (2015). Sleep Deprivation. *Obstetrics and gynecology clinics of North America, 42*(3), 493–506. https://doi.org/10.1016/j.ogc.2015.05.013

Powermove: Minimize EMF

Remove or unplug all electronic devices from your sleeping area or disable their Wi-Fi feature to reduce EMF exposure. If you want to go extreme, sleep in a faraday cage as Matt does.

25 - The lighting we use in our homes can damage our health.

"'Our study revealed that the response of healthy skin cells to UV emitted from CFL bulbs is consistent with damage from ultraviolet radiation,' said Professor Rafailovich. 'Skin cell damage was further enhanced when low dosages of TiO2 nanoparticles were introduced to the skin cells prior to exposure.'"

Powermove: Remove Toxic Lighting

Get rid of all the fluorescent lights in your home and office. Opt for full-spectrum light in places where you need traditional lighting and red light for places where you sleep whenever possible.

Toxins Are Unavoidable in Today's World

There are over 15,000 new man-made chemicals that the human organism hasn't evolved enough in order to deal with. We don't know what the real risks are. Are you going to wait another 20 years to find out what the health consequences are?

A simple truth is, toxins impair optimal biological function.

Don't let the mind-opening facts inside this chapter scare you. This is a small list of the potential toxic threats that are around us. The first step is to develop awareness ***without fear***. There is no need for fear. Fear creates its own toxins by elevating cortisol, epinephrine, and norepinephrine.

The key is to make one small change at a time. Improve your water supply... Get rid of plastics from your kitchen... buy organic foods, etc...

It's virtually impossible to eliminate all toxins because there are so many of them. You would have to move into a pristine jungle where man has never visited before and eat off the land. Probably not gonna happen. Our approach is to gently remove them from the body and to optimize the cellular environment.

We are not treating disease. Our approach helps your body return to its natural state and do its own healing. Your body is the ultimate detoxification machine. Of course, we can help it by giving it the right nutrients such as enzymes.

To recap, we don't want you to get lost inside of all the toxins and chemicals, because it's a negative-based focus. Being aware of the obstacles is important, but overly focusing on the problem or developing a paranoid psychology is self-destructive. Instead put your energy on positive, proactive solutions like the Powermoves in this chapter and throughout the book.

Chapter 5

Biological Enemy #4: The 5 Deadly Deficiencies

In this chapter, you will learn:

- **Is your diet or supplement stack leaving you without critical vitamins and minerals?**

- Why addressing "deficiency" is NOT enough for fully bioptimized health.

- **How you can essentially be deficient in protein — even when you consume lots of protein...**

- And much more...

Deficiency

Deadly Deficiency #1: Minerals and Vitamins

Here's how deficiency is traditionally defined: *In medicine, a deficiency is a lack or shortage of a functional entity, by less than normal or necessary supply or function.* [124]

What is the basic nutrient amount that prevents one from getting disease?

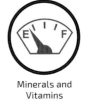

Minerals and
Vitamins

The early research was with sailors. They discovered that when they were on long journeys, they would get a condition called scurvy. Scurvy was caused by a lack of vitamin C. So eventually they started adding lemons and limes onto boats.

At that time, medical research began to discover the minimum amount to prevent the development of a given disease.

Eventually, this led to the development of the RDA (Recommended Daily Allowance). For instance, how much iron did you need to prevent anemia?

How much vitamin D do you need to prevent osteoporosis?

How much vitamin C to prevent scurvy?

Doctors and scientists have figured out that many of the obvious diseases stem from a lack of major vitamins and minerals.

To illustrate our current state of deficiency, take a look at what was published in Scientific American in 2011, with regards to the vitamin content of the food we consume:

---

[124] *Deficiency.* TheFreeDictionary.com. (2007). Retrieved 2 October 2020, from http://medical-dictionary.thefreedictionary.com/deficiency.

"A Kushi Institute analysis of nutrient data from 1975 to 1997 found that average calcium levels in 12 fresh vegetables dropped 27 percent; iron levels 37 percent; vitamin A levels 21 percent, and vitamin C levels 30 percent. A similar study of British nutrient data from 1930 to 1980, published in the British Food Journal, found that in 20 vegetables the average calcium content had declined 19 percent; iron 22 percent; and potassium 14 percent."

This is thought to be a result of modern-day agricultural practices, which are decreasing the soil quality used to grow our food.

Magnesium for example, has an impact on mental health. It works on over 300 different functions in the body. That's why we created the world's first 7 magnesium formula called Magnesium Breakthrough.

Calcium is essential for the strength of your bones. Zinc is required for vitamin transportation. Iron is required for oxygen to get to your cells.

If we're not getting these minerals from our food, we have to get them from somewhere else, if we want to become biologically optimized.

Dr. Linus Pauling, Dr. Abram Hoffer, and Dr. David Hawkins published a book called Orthomolecular Psychiatry, in the early 70s.

These doctors had developed megadose vitamin and mineral protocols to treat advanced states of medical illness like schizophrenia.

Although many traditional scientists and doctors refuted their work, thousands of people from around the world poured into their clinics for treatment. Many of these patients came from some of the most affluent families in the world who had tried everything with their ill family members.

Oftentimes these clients were completely healed by using mega doses of various nutrients, eliminating sugar and chemical toxins.

Here's the critical question that we are focused on:

What's the optimum vitamin and mineral dosage for super health or as we call it BiOptimized Health?

Over the last few decades, most medical practitioners have been focusing on symptom management through pharmaceutical drugs.
Let's consider for a moment what deficiency is from a BiOptimized perspective.

If you take a pro-athlete, a 27-year-old pregnant woman, and an 80-year-old grandma... Do you think their mineral and vitamin requirements are going to be different?

They've got completely different lifestyles, genetics, physical capacities, energy requirements, and goals.

Yet remarkably, many nutrition schools, universities, and so-called "experts" cling to the outdated beliefs that requirements are generally similar for most adults.

They have no differentiation in requirements between the individuals.

The appropriate levels of bioavailable minerals and vitamins are essential for optimizing your health based on your lifestyle, activity, goals, and genetics.

Aim to get as much of the micronutrients you need from food. However, it's almost impossible to get the necessary amounts due to the modern farm and food production processes. This is where supplements come in.

That's why we created Primergen V and Primergen-M. These formulas give your cells almost all of the critical vitamins and nutrients they need to operate at their best.

Deadly Deficiency #2: Enzymes

According to Dr. Edward Howell, author of the book Enzyme Nutrition, enzymes have both a biochemical and biological function. Enzymes are the bridge between inorganic matter and organic living tissue.

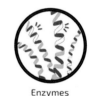

Enzymes

Enzymes are required for virtually every single metabolic and biochemical function in the body, and there are literally thousands of different enzymes in the body. Dr. Hiromi Shinya estimates the number of enzymatic reactions in the body at 25,000.

Every time you think a thought, blink an eye, or flex a muscle — enzymes are involved.

Dr. Howell first got turned onto the idea of enzymes around 70 years ago after reading a shocking study performed by Dr. Pottenger with cats. This experiment revealed the severe negative consequences of an enzyme deficient diet.

In this experiment, Dr. Pottenger fed one group of cats an enzyme deficient diet (cooked food), and another group of cats ate enzyme-rich foods.

In all cases, the cats fed the enzyme deficient diet developed diseases sooner, died earlier, and passed on various mutations to their offspring.

By the third generation of cats, the genetic disease became widespread. There was an inability to procreate, and unusual social behavior, such as eating their young.

These findings were later replicated by Dr. Howell with an array of animals. He saw similar results, outlined in his books Enzyme Nutrition and Enzymes for Health and Longevity. This has profound implications and applications to humans because most people's diets have almost no enzymes. Why?

Every time you cook food with heat higher than 114F (41 C), all enzymes in the food die. Every time a food is sprayed with pesticides, fungicides, and herbicides — the enzymes in the food die. Every time you eat cooked food, you need to use your own body's enzyme supply to digest the food into utilizable biomaterials.

So the only way to get enzymes in a diet is to eat organic, raw food. This isn't feasible for most people.

Your body has a limited amount of enzymes, often referred to as the enzyme potential. According to Dr. Howell, "the length of life is inversely related to the enzyme potential of the organisms".

Loosely translated, this means the more enzymes you have in the body, the longer you can live, and the more capacity your body has to perform biochemical functions.

What's fascinating is longevity studies have shown a correlation between eating less and longer lifespan.

Could it be that consuming less food preserves the body's enzyme reserves? Dr. Howell certainly seemed to think so.

How does this relate to Biological Optimization?

Let's look at athletes and people who are looking to build strength, increase muscle mass, or operate at peak physical performance levels. These individuals tend to consume massive amounts of cooked protein, processed protein, whey protein, and casein protein.

They're eating all these proteins that have zero enzymes in them.

Virtually every time they consume protein, they're asking their bodies to produce protease to digest the food (proteases digest protein to amino acids).

Athletes who consume large amounts of enzyme deficient protein often end up with digestive issues because they don't have enough enzymes to break down the protein.

Athletes often increase protein consumption more and more because they believe it helps them recover from their workouts.

Over time, the high levels of protein consumption drain the enzymatic reserves and compromise the body's abilities to get nutrients from their food.

Athletes often start using steroids to counteract the catabolic effects of their training and diets.

The answer is to consume the right enzymes for your diet.

For example, if you're on a ketogenic diet, we suggest kApex. It's loaded with lipases that break down fats into usable fatty acids. Then, the L-carnitine transports those fatty acids into the mitochondria and then we boost the mitochondria with several ingredients. The result? Way more energy and no digestive issues on a high-fat diet.

If you're on a paleo diet or any high-protein diet, we suggest taking MassZymes. It's the strongest proteolytic enzyme on the market today. It will help you get a lot more valuable amino acids from the food you eat.

We've also created special enzymes for specific needs. For example, gluten is a protein that is very difficult for the body to break down and creates inflammation. There is one enzyme that does the job and it's called DPP-IV (Dipeptidyl peptidase-4). That's the key enzyme we use in Gluten Guardian.

We will go into greater depth on enzymes in Chapter 9, Biological Optimizer #1: Nutrification, BiOptimizing Conversion Of Food Into Nutrients.

Deadly Deficiency #3: Probiotics

Probiotics (means pro-life) are bacteria that are essential to life. In fact, they were amongst the first life forms on Earth.

Probiotics

Every person on the planet has trillions of bacteria inside them, which digest food, create vitamins and other vital immune system factors.

Probiotics are the keystone of your immune system. They are the first line of defense against viruses, bugs, and flus. They create a shield within your intestinal tract that stops the bad guys dead in their tracks.

Probiotics have been linked in research to easier weight loss, anti-depression effects, and more.

Probiotics have been used for thousands of years in optimizing health functions.

We get them from organic foods that haven't been cooked and fermented foods.

In chapter 4, we revealed how antibiotics wipe out good and bad bacteria strains. Then foreign invaders can easily get a hold of your digestive system and create havoc.

The other challenge these unfriendly organisms create is, they make it harder for "good strains" to reclaim the terrain. Often people pound even more antibiotics to counterattack these bad strains, which further upsets the body's health.

Unfortunately because of the consumption of cooked food and overload of toxins in people's lives - many people are severely deficient in good probiotics in their gut biome.

There are thousands of different strains of bacteria. Some are destructive for your health and some very good for you. The goal is to increase the good guys and diminish the bad guys.

One of the best ways to change your gut biome is to change your diet. Each strain of bacteria lives off of certain foods. If someone eats Doritos and donuts daily, then the strains that live off of sugar and processed foods will thrive. If you eat carnivore style, then the strains that feed on meat will grow in population. If you follow a plant-based diet, then the strains that love plants will thrive.

This is why an "elimination diet" can fix gut dysbiosis. By shifting to a carnivore diet or a plant-based diet, you will starve many strains including the ones that may be causing problems.

Another keynote related to this is food cravings. The majority of your food cravings come from the bacteria in your gut sending signals to your brain to feed them. So when you change diets, expect cravings for a few days. The good news is, as you feed your body new foods consistently your cravings will shift to your new diet.

We suggest supplementing with Biome Breakthrough. It will help rebuild the biofilm in your gut as well as eliminate bad bacteria that could be creating problems.

We also recommend using P3OM, a patented strain of L Plantarum OM. In the patent, it's been shown to be anti-viral, anti-retroviral, anti-tumoral, and proteolytic (which means it helps break down protein into usable amino acids like enzymes).

The good news is, it's relatively easy to fix this problem once you know how.

Deadly Deficiency #4: Amino Acids

Amino acids are the building blocks of protein and proteins are the engines of life. Most of your organs and muscles are made of amino acids. The neurotransmitters that create your brain's reality are made of amino acids. Your body makes over 7,000 critical amino acid combinations called peptides. Your body combines the twenty types of amino acids in the body which signals and activates thousands of critical functions in your body.

Amino Acids

There are 2 potential dangers with proteins and amino acids:

1 - An overload of undigested proteins
2 - An amino acid deficiency

First, let's discuss the overload problem.

Over the last few decades, "protein" has been one of the biggest selling supplements. However, it's not PROTEIN that matters, it's the amino acids. You can eat hundreds of grams of protein a day, and waste your hard-earned money. Unless you're breaking the protein down into amino acids, transporting those amino acids through the intestinal tract, and then assimilating them into your body, they're useless and even dangerous.

An undigested protein is a serious toxin. Many deadly allergic reactions are caused by undigested proteins that the body identifies as an "allergen" and then the immune system overreacts in order to combat it.

But the dangers don't end there. Here's an excerpt from The Longevity Code by Kris Verburgh[125] as he discusses the long term problems of too much protein:

"As the decades pass, they (the cells) become so stuffed with clumps of proteins that they can no longer function— they age and ultimately they die.

A similar process occurs in the brain. One of the most feared aging-related diseases is Alzheimer's disease. There are several forms of dementia; the most common is Alzheimer's, which occurs in 65 percent of dementia cases. Alzheimer's disease is caused by proteins that accumulate both in and around brain cells. In the long term, the brain cells are literally smothered by this agglomeration of proteins and they die. Once about a quarter of the approximately 86 billion brain cells have disappeared that way, people develop the first signs of Alzheimer's: forgetfulness.

Research has shown that supercentenarians often die of a disease we call amyloidosis. Some researchers even believe that 70 percent of deaths of supercentenarians is due to amyloidosis. This is actually a generalized agglomeration of proteins everywhere in the body. One type of protein in particular clusters in the body and causes extensive damage; namely, transthyretin."

Undigested proteins can create digestive distress in the intestinal tract.

After scoping 370,000 colons over his career, Dr. Hiromi Shinya, who was the leading colon doctor in the world, found that almost all of the cancer patients he dealt with, had massive quantities of putrid, undigested meat and dairy inside their intestinal tracts.

Based on these disgusting discoveries, we can safely assume that most people aren't absorbing 100% of the protein they're consuming.

Most athletes are advised by nutritionists to consume 0.7 to 1 gram of protein per pound of bodyweight.

For someone who weighs 200 lbs, their target would be 140 to 200 grams of protein a day.

What's happening with all this protein if most can't be digested without enzymes?

Is it possible that it's contributing to the rise in colon cancer?

I'll let you make your own conclusion.

What's the solution to this problem? It's simple: proteolytic enzymes. Proteases are the specific enzymes that break down proteins into usable amino acids.

---

125 Verburgh, K., & Vonhof, T. *The longevity code.* (2018)

Now let's shift to amino acid deficiencies.

Amino acid deficiency is one of the leading causes of the gradual muscle loss that happens after people turn 28.

Why is this happening?

1 -   A steady decrease in HCL (stomach acid).
2 -   A decline in the body's enzyme production.

Powermove: Take HCL and Proteolytic Enzymes

The answer to this problem is simple: consume HCL and proteolytic enzymes with each meal. This is an important digestive optimization practice as people get into their 30s and beyond. We suggest taking 1-2 caps of HCL (such as HCL Breakthrough) along with 2-5 caps of proteolytic enzymes such as MassZymes with each meal. Your digestion will transform as a result.

By the time most people turn 60 and 70, there is a massive drop in strength and lean muscle. Often this can lead to catastrophic accidents that could have easily been avoided with stronger muscles.

The point is: we're severely overestimating how much usable protein we're actually digesting and absorbing.

We'll reveal how to reverse this problem in chapter 8.

Deadly Deficiency #5: Water

Dehydration may be the biggest enemy to optimized physical and mental performance.

Water

"Many people think they get plenty of fluids on a daily basis. What they don't realize, however, is that they may be dehydrated which could lead to a slew of health issues including fatigue, joint pain, and weight gain.

Most people know that they are supposed to drink water, but up to 75 percent of Americans may be functioning in a chronic state of dehydration, according to new research.

We have a tendency in the U.S. to drink a lot of beverages that are mildly dehydrating, said Mary Grace Webb,

Assistant Director for Clinical Nutrition at New York Hospital." [126]

The human body is approximately 75% water. This water is separated into two distinct categories. Fluid outside the cells, such as the blood, and fluid inside the cells, which maintain the cell rigidity and function.

Both are critical to optimal health and performance. Over the last two or three decades, there has been tremendous misinformation on hydration and performance.

Wade has researched hundreds of experts in the field of hydration, and all experts agree that hydration is a critical factor in optimal health, nutrient absorption, and toxin elimination.

Dr. Peter Agre won a Nobel prize for his work on demonstrating how protein chains act as a gate on the cells of your body. These channels let water in and out depending on the size of the molecule, osmotic pressure, pH, and charge of the water.

The channels play a key role in whether a liquid hydrates you or dehydrates you at a cellular level.

We have personally tested the majority of the water technologies on the market.

7 Critical Factors You Need to Know About Water

I.   *It's best not to consume water with chlorine, fluoride, or chloramine in it. Removing these contaminants from your water is important. Many plastic water bottle companies add fluoride to the water, which has been shown to have a variety of physiological impairing effects. Especially in thyroid metabolism (which can impact your body fat levels) and pineal gland function.*

II.   *Bottled water contains plastics that lead to increased levels of xenoestrogens in the body. These contribute to birth defects, low sperm count, and other diseases. There's a documentary called "The Disappearing Male" that dives deep into this.*

III.   *Reverse Osmosis (RO) water is great for getting contaminants out of water but tends to have a negative effect on pH, energy levels, and long term health. If you currently use RO water, be sure to add organic minerals (such as Primergen-M) to replace the lost minerals.*

IV.   *Most municipalities fail basic water safety parameters. Most of the government regulations are over 35 years old. A recent White Paper suggests the US government would have to spend 1 trillion dollars on its water systems to upgrade to acceptable health standards put forth by water experts.*

V.   *High pH Ionized water penetrates the cells 6 times faster than tap water or bottled water, according to nuclear resonance imaging shown to me by Harvard Medical Vascular Surgeon Dr. Horst Filtzer.*

---

[126] *Seen At 11: Drinking More Water Could Make You Feel A Lot Better.* Newyork.cbslocal.com. (2013). Retrieved 2 October 2020, from https://newyork.cbslocal.com/2013/06/07/seen-at-11-drinking-more-water-could-be-the-cure-for-some-serious-ailments/.

VI.   By passing water through electrical currents, you can alter water to serve as a powerful antioxidant by increasing donor electrons that pick up free radicals. You can also create water that can kill viruses, bacteria, and other harmful pathogens. You can alter the water to emulsify oil, tone skin, or to remove pesticides from food.

VII. The "normal" recommended amount of water is 8 glasses a day (which is 2 liters). However, if you're an active person, or you live in hot climates, you need far more than this. For people aiming for peak performance, 4 to 6 liters of water consumption per day is sufficient enough water to maintain hydration, assuming the water is devoid of chemicals. For optimal levels, we suggest using a medical-grade ionizer hooked to your tap with the appropriate pre-filters installed, based on your municipality's water contaminants. We also suggest consuming the water fresh or keeping it sealed in dark amber glass bottles to retain charge, pH, and freshness of water.

Water Powermoves:

1 - Avoid Plastic Bottles

Avoid plastic bottles as much as possible. Try using glass bottles to avoid absorbing plastics. Bottle water in the sun is even more dangerous as the plastic leaches up to 8X faster.[127]

2 - Mineralize Your Water

Adding ¼ to ½ tsp of high-quality salts (we recommend Himalayan or sea salt) is an inexpensive way to get more minerals into your body. The sodium will help you absorb the water more.

For people on ketogenic diets, we also recommend adding ½ tsp of cream of tartar with the salt in 2 liters of water once a day to get the necessary amounts of potassium. We also recommend using 3 droppers a day of Primergen-M to get the necessary amounts of trace minerals.

3 - Avoid Tap Water

As mentioned in a previous Powermove, use powerful whole house water filters.

---

[127] Westerhoff, P., Prapaipong, P., Shock, E., & Hillaireau, A. (2008). Antimony leaching from polyethylene terephthalate (PET) plastic used for bottled drinking water. *Water research, 42*(3), 551–556. https://doi.org/10.1016/j.watres.2007.07.048

Over the last 7 years, we have developed an optimal intensive hydration protocol that allows virtually anyone suffering from chronic dehydration to optimize their body's hydration, intracellular, and extracellular fluid levels.

I have also found that ionized water from a medical-grade ionization (look for ISO 13485 Certification) device hydrates your body faster than any other beverage. It reduces delayed onset muscle soreness, free radicals in the blood, and boosts your energy. Now you understand why people's health, energy, and body fat levels continue to plummet for the past few decades.

Don't let these new revelations worry you. In the next 3 chapters, you'll discover the simple solutions that can reverse and fix these deficiencies and remove toxins.

PART 2: THE SOLUTION

Now we're going to shift into the solution.

What are the critical things that have the most impact on your aesthetics, health, and performance?

First, we will redefine what nutrition really means. Most people think that nutrition is just eating good food. It's far more than this. We will reveal the 3 phases of Nutrification and how to optimize all 5 stages of digestion. The chapters are loaded with practice nutritional advice.

Then, we will reveal how to take your sleep quality to a new dimension. The positive effects of high-quality sleep are life-changing.

Then we will cover the unexpected benefits of building lean muscle mass and lowering body fat. The benefits aren't just looking your best, but they are the keys to maximizing your lifespan and healthspan.

In chapter 14, we dive into one of the most overlooked aspects of health: optimizing the nervous system.

Want to keep your mind sharp and productive and maintain your mental prime? Chapter 15 has the answers.

Then we reveal the mindblowing benefits of heliotherapy. It boosts virtually every aspect of your health.

Then we wrap up by discussing the future of health. And we finish what we think is the most important chapter: the Biological Optimization process.

The Appendixes are loaded with gold too. Appendix A reveals the protocols that we use with our clients to deliver world-class results.

Appendix B gives you the guide to building your own team of health experts to mentor you along your journey.

Chapter 6

Biological Optimizer #1: Getting Into Your Optimal Nutrient Zone

"Sola dosis facit venenum" translation: *"The dose makes the poison"*
- Paracelsus

In this chapter, you will learn:

- **The 5 levels of nutrification and the "sweet spot" for optimum performance.**

- How to dial in all your key nutrient levels and feel amazing.

- **The best testing methods to determine and reverse any deficiencies.**

- And much more...

When it comes to nutrients there are 2 ways it can kill us:

1 - Long term deficiencies.
2 - Deadly overloads.[128]

Dosage Spectrum

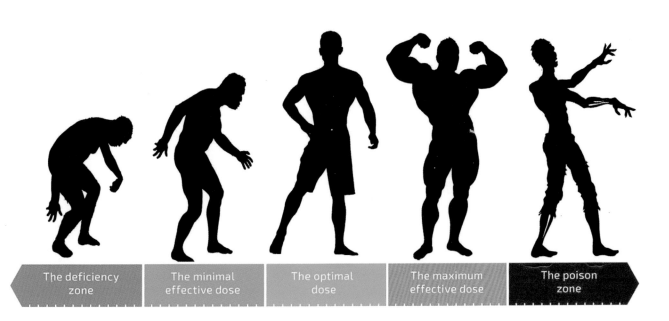

The deficiency zone | The minimal effective dose | The optimal dose | The maximum effective dose | The poison zone

---

[128] *Drank too much water, woman dies.* The Globe and Mail. (2017). Retrieved 2 October 2020, from https://www.theglobeand-mail.com/news/world/drank-too-much-water-woman-dies/article1069137/.

Here's a critical BiOptimization lesson, for almost every nutrient there is:

1 -   The deficiency zone.
2 -   The minimal effective dose.
3 -   The optimal dose.
4 -   The maximum effective dose.
5 -   The deadly poison zone.

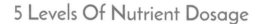

5 Levels Of Nutrient Dosage

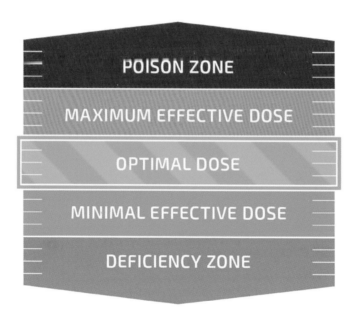

The Deficiency Zone

The deficiency zone is where there aren't enough nutrients for your body to operate at its peak and diseases and other health problems occur. This can create a cascade of secondary negative effects.

Here's an analogy to illustrate what we mean. When Matt was 16 years old, his father's car had transmission problems. His father said, *"Don't go anywhere with the car, we need to fix the transmission. It could damage the engine."*

Well, Matt being young, ignorant, and stubborn decided to go see his girlfriend who lived /30 miles away. On the way back, the car was stuck on the 2nd gear and the RPMs were maxed out the entire drive. By the time he got home, he had cooked the engine and it was completely destroyed. His father wasn't a happy camper.

The point of this story is, when one system gets compromised it affects other systems. This can create dire consequences.

We already discussed some of the biggest deficiencies in a previous chapter.

The Minimal Effective Dose

Most people are in this zone with the majority of the body's critical nutrients. In this trange, the body has some of the nutrients, but not enough to operate at its best.

One of the problems of being in this zone is that over time, it's easy to slip into the deficiency zone. As we age, a lot of our body's functions decline. We tend to absorb fewer nutrients and our ability to assimilate them gets weaker as we highlighted in the Aging chapter.

Take digestion for an example. As we age, our body's enzyme reserves get depleted. We produce less stomach acid. This means we absorb fewer nutrients including critical amino acids. What are some of the consequences? Your body produces fewer neuro-transmitters, which is vital for your brain to operate at its peak and feel happy. Your muscles lack amino acids, which leads to muscle loss. Loss of muscle leads to a slower metabolism and other negative issues.

The Optimal Dose

There is an optimal zone where you're giving your body the appropriate amount of nutrients for it to operate at its best.

And we're not just talking about macronutrients (carbs, proteins, and fats). We're talking about everything: micronutrients, enzymes, probiotics, phytonutrients, etc...

The goal is to get each of your body's nutrients and hormones into the optimal zone. This is easier said than done.

There are many considerations to figure this out:

- Your age: The older you get, the harder it is to absorb nutrients.

- Your lean body mass: The more you have, the more you need.

- Your metabolism: Some people utilize nutrients at a much faster rate.

- Your genetics: This is one of the most significant ones because genetic mutations (which everyone has) can cause deficiencies.

- Lifestyle: Are you drinking, partying, and eating garbage? Are you working 80 hours a week? Are you sleeping enough?

- Exercise: Do you think an Olympian who trains 12 times a week needs more nutrients than someone who watched 40 hours of Netflix a week?

And here are 3 problems that most of us face:

1 - Lack of good data
2 - Lack of visibility
3 - Lack of knowledge

Lack of good, convenient data can be solved for the most part with blood, urine, and saliva tests. However, this leads to the second problem that all of us have...

Lack of visibility over certain biological systems is a big challenge. There are many things that we don't have tests for yet. The good news is, hundreds of companies are working hard to create better tests and data for us to use.

Lack of knowledge is essentially ignorance. There are things that we don't know that we don't know. The body is incredibly complex and we're still figuring things out. The great news is, health knowledge is expanding exponentially.

Powermove: Get Regular Blood Work and Other Tests

It's crucial as a BiOptimizer, to get blood work on a regular basis. We suggest every 6 months and if you can afford it, every 3 months.

Other tests that are valuable include genetics, gut health tests, and hormone tests.

We're also big proponents of using biofeedback devices such as the Oura ring and fitness trackers.

Problems with the RDA

Here's one of the bigger challenges: we're still learning what the optimal dose is for most nutrients. The RDA stands for the recommended daily allowance. There are 2 standards.

The first was produced by the FDA and hasn't been updated since 1968! They gave the world a simplified estimation of nutrient needs based on a 2,000 calorie diet regardless of age, sex, or pregnancy.

The second set is produced by the Institute of Medicine. These numbers are reasonably precise because they're broken down by age and sex, and they're updated fairly often. Those numbers give us:

- Recommended Dietary Allowance (RDA): an estimation of how much of a nutrient you need, based on your age, sex, and pregnancy status.

- Adequate Intake (AI): how much of a nutrient you need to avoid an obvious deficiency disease.

- Tolerable Upper Limit (UL): how much of a nutrient you can safely take without overdose.

The problems with the RDA and DRI (daily recommended intake) is that it doesn't factor your genetics, your goals, and other personal factors.

There's a lot missing if you want to become a Biologically Optimized Human. That's why you should keep educating yourself and learning.

The field of health, fitness, and nutrition is evolving by the day. Hold all knowledge as provisional because new knowledge makes old knowledge obsolete. This is also why you want to build a Jedi Council of health experts that are guiding you on your mission.

The Maximum Effective Dose

Beyond Biological Optimization is maximization. This is where the goal is to achieve the most extreme results possible.

Professional bodybuilders are the perfect example: their goal is to build as much muscle and lose as much body fat as humanly possible. They're going above and beyond any genetic limit set. That's why they use extreme doses of testosterone, SARMS, GH, and other drugs to achieve their goals.

Professional athletes in general operate the Maximization Zone. Their goal is maximum speed, maximum power, maximum endurance, or maximum performance.

They're willing to sacrifice the health side of the BiOptimization Triangle to achieve their goals.

The sports researcher Robert Goldman polled 198 world-class athletes, asking: *"Would you take a pill, that would guarantee a gold medal even if you knew that it would kill you in five years?"'* **More than half said they'd do it.** In other words, they want athletic success and they want that gold medal more than they want life itself.

Even many purpose-driven entrepreneurs fall into this category. They're on a mission and they're willing to sacrifice their health to get there.

First of all, we applaud the dedication and drive of these people. They're a special breed that are extremely driven to become the best at what they do.

Our message is, you can achieve even better levels of success by focusing on the health side of the BiOptimization Triangle. Longer careers and even better performance can be achieved by optimizing vs. maximizing.

Short term, the body can tolerate short bouts of maximization. The key is to cycle periods of recovery with these intense bursts. Similar to an engine, it can tolerate redlining the RPMs for short periods of time, but if you redline it too long you'll cook the engine (like Matt did).

The Poison Zone

Virtually every substance has an LD50 which means the Median Lethal Dose. It means the lethal dose of a substance would kill 50% of the population.

On the extreme side, the deadliest toxin in the world, botulinum, kills a human at 1 nanogram per kilogram.

Everything at the right dose can kill us including water. There was a lady who drank 10 liters of water who died. This is a bit misleading because it's a mineral deficiency that killed her. When you drink water, it pulls minerals out of your body. Some waters like distilled water, aggressively eliminate crucial minerals and can create serious health issues including death.

Our advice is to be mindful of the LD50 of the supplements and other nutrients that you take.

Conclusion

The goal is to get your body into the Optimal Nutrient Zone and keep it there. In order to do this, consistent, frequent testing is required.

Chapter 7

Biological Optimizer #1: The 3 Nutrification Phases

In this chapter, you will learn:

- **What plants can teach us about multiplying and optimizing nutrient absorption.**

- How to assure the nutrients you consume from food and supplements don't go to waste.

- **3 phases of getting nutrients INTO your cells and the dangers of missing even 1 phase.**

- And much more...

Most of the information in the dietary world, inside of medical research, focuses on raw materials. *"You need this much vitamin D, this much protein, this many carbohydrates, and this many fats."*

However, just as important as the raw materials are the bio-workers. ***Inside the body, the only workers are enzymes and probiotics.*** They do the work of virtually every metabolic, digestive, and immune system process.

Imagine, you're building your dream home and you order all of the finest raw materials. You've got Italian marble, bricks, mortar, cement, mixers, Elon Musk's solar roofing tiles, exotic woods, but you've got no workers. Will your house get built? Obviously not.

They're essentially inert substances and they require workers to put them together.

Keep reading to gain a comprehensive understanding of how enzymes and probiotics play a significant role in optimizing your biological state.

The Three Phases to Nutrification

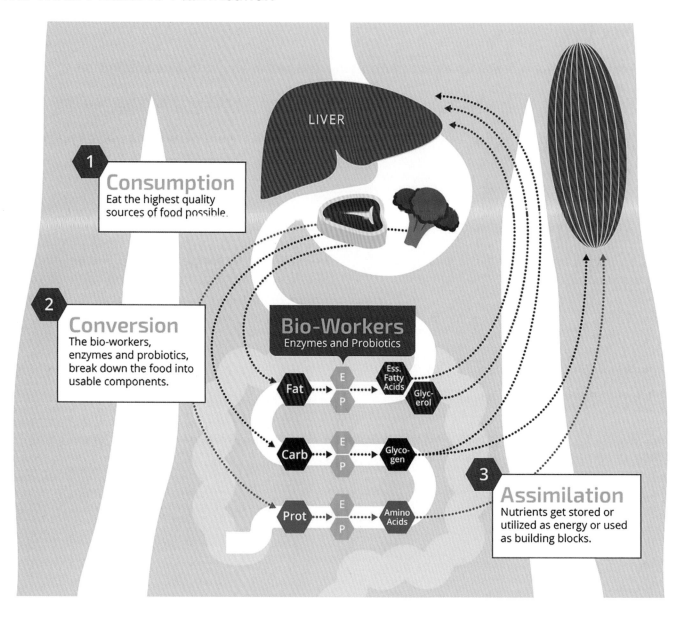

We define nutrification as the process of consuming foods, breaking them down into usable components, transporting them into your bloodstream, and then assimilating those components in the body.

Step 1: Consumption

In this stage, we flood your digestive system with the essential nutrients required for you to achieve your health and performance goals based on your genetics. We have developed these principles based on Two Time Nobel Prize Winner Dr. Linus Pauling's research on Orthomolecular Nutrition. We call it the "plant theory of nutrification."

The Plant Theory of Nutrification

Imagine your body is a beautiful glorious plant.

For a plant to be strong and hardy, it needs an optimal mix of soil (probiotics and minerals), sun (vitamins), water, and enzymes (innate in the seed).

When the plant lacks any of these, it suffers.

When the plant has too much water it can drown. When it has too much sun, it can dry out. If it has too many minerals, it can kill the plant. Once the pot is full of the raw ingredients you simply optimize your intake to match your burn rate.

Your body is the same. It needs the optimal levels of oxygen, water, proteins, fats, carbohydrates, minerals, vitamins, enzymes, and probiotics to rock and roll.

The goal of phase 1 is to give your body all the highest quality nutrients it needs to be at its best. This is where buying the best real food possible matters. Buy organic vegetables and fruits if possible. Buying heirlooms vegetables is even better. When you buy meat, focus on grass-fed. Even better, eat wild game.

How much should you eat? This is where your weight, age, personal lifestyle, genetics, and goals need to be factored. Doing blood work and genetic tests are critical to find if you have mutations that are causing deficiencies.

Athletes have a higher burn rate than someone who's sedentary. They're exhausting their resources at a faster rate.

If you're looking to gain maximum muscle mass, we'd be focusing on enzymes and protein.

If you're looking to burn fat, we'd probably be looking at increases in protein, probiotics, vitamins, and minerals.

If you're traveling a lot, we'd probably be focused a little bit more on the probiotics to enhance your immunity.

If you have too many heavy metals in your body, we'll go on a healthy detox phase.

In the consumption stage, we give your body all the macronutrients it needs including live plant proteins, essential fatty acids, organic protein sources, phytonutrients, and therapeutic levels of vitamins and minerals.

Step 2: Conversion

The second step to optimize your digestion is to extract nutrients from the food you're currently getting.

This involves increasing our "bio-workers": enzymes and probiotics.

These are the "workers" who do all the work as far as deconstructing the food into its raw components. They deconstruct protein into usable amino acids, fats into fatty acids, and carbs into glycogen. They're also involved in clearing out toxins from your body.

Enzymes enhance your body's ability to move toxins out of the body, and more importantly, rebuild tissues that have been damaged from chemical toxins and oxidative stress.

Most formulations of various enzymes are made up of amylase, lipase, and protease.

They break down your carbohydrates, fats, and proteins respectively.

If you're looking to build muscle mass, you need to shunt more amino acids into the cells where it can be used to build muscle.

Wade has been able to maintain a body weight of 200 lbs as a vegetarian eating 75 grams to 100 grams of protein a day using MassZymes. The evidence is showing that we're able to maintain high levels of muscle mass on very low protein diets because of the efficiency of the bio-workers.

We're able to get more out of the protein we're consuming and subject ourselves to less oxidative stress.

Probiotics are organisms that break down food even further, help fight off bad bacteria and viruses, remove toxic garbage, and run an incredible array of biological functions for digestion. They also produce neurotransmitters, immune factors, vitamins, enzymes, and many other critical nutrients for the body.

They're one of the best weapons to protect your immunity and maintain optimal digestive function.

Virtually all of our clients consume powerful probiotics and enzymes on a daily basis to help them detox and perform at their highest capacity, day in and day out.

Think of the enzymes as a lawnmower and the probiotics as the lawn mulcher. Together, they deconstruct food into the fuel and building blocks your body needs to be BiOptimized.

Step 3: Assimilation

Assimilation is the final step of nutrification. The amino acids, fatty acids, and glycogen cross the intestinal barrier and enter the bloodstream.

In this final step, amino acids become assimilated as muscle, organs, neurotransmitters, and peptides. Guess what actually does the work? Enzymes. Again, enzymes do over 25,000 different functions in the body. Enzymes are the workers that do the assimilation.

Fatty acids become either energy, brain matter, body fat, myelin sheath, hormones, and many other things. What does the work? Enzymes.

Glycogen gets stored either in the liver, muscle, or turns into body fat via the gluconeogenesis process. Gluconeogenesis is a 25 cent word that means, you didn't burn the excess carbs so we're going to store it as fat.

The key to optimizing assimilation is keeping your body's enzyme reserves high.

Other keys are minerals such as magnesium. Magnesium is involved in over 300 of the body's functions. Magnesium helps optimize many of these assimilation processes.
Giving your cells all the micronutrients it needs is critical. Micronutrients include all the big minerals and trace minerals.

Then you use your biofeedback, blood work, and other health analysis to optimize your nutritional choices and supplements even more precisely. This is a core part of the Biological Optimization process.

In summary, the 3 nutrification phases are:

1 - Consumption: consume the highest quality food possible.
2 - Conversion: consume enzymes, probiotics, and HCL to maximize the breakdown of the food.
3 - Assimilation: consume plenty of enzymes that help assist your body's assimilation process.

We're going to go deeper into each one of these steps in the following chapters.

Chapter 8

Biological Optimizer #1: Nutrification, BiOptimizing Your Consumption

In this chapter, you will learn:

- **Are you getting the right macros for your body? Here's how to know.**

- 6 ways to avoid picking the wrong protein and never wasting money.

- **Why even the best "good fats" aren't good for some people.**

- And much more...

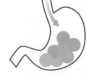

Consumption

Phase number one is consumption. What you eat. What goes in your mouth. This is when you add the essential raw components into the system.

Your goal is to give your body all of the macronutrients and micronutrients in the right quantities and qualities that it needs to function optimally. This includes conductive minerals, bioavailable vitamins, phytonutrients, amino acids, essential fatty acids, enzymes, and probiotics.

We'll divide this chapter into 2 sections: *macro-nutrification* and *micro-nutrification*.

Macro Nutrification: Protein and Essential Fatty Acids

Your body needs amino acids and essential fatty acids to survive and thrive. Amino acids are obtained from the protein. Essential fatty acids are obtained from fats.

As we discussed earlier, amino acids rebuild muscle tissue, peptides, neurotransmitters, organs, and much more.

Your body also requires essential fatty acids to build hormones and rebuild organs and provide structure to other tissues.

Those are the 2 most vital macro-nutrients your body needs.

Yes, your body uses carbohydrates for energy, however, we can assure you that there's no lack of carbohydrates missing in most people's diets. You can stop eating carbohydrates and your body will switch over to using fat for energy. It will convert the fats (including body fat) into ketones.

Selecting the Best Proteins for Your Body

As far as consuming proteins, organic or wild meats and fish are ideal. One key when choosing proteins is to avoid or minimize inflammatory proteins. For many people, A1 protein coming from the majority of dairy products coming from cows can be inflammatory. Better dairy options are from sheep, goats, bison, etc.

Other proteins to avoid are from processed meats.[129] [130] [131] Processed meats contain more advanced glycation end products (AGEs) than most other meats. They are caused by cooking the meat at high temperatures. These accumulate in the body and eventually stop cells from functioning.

As far as selecting the best proteins for your body, looking at your gut biome is another powerful tool. Gut biome tests can help detect the bacteria you have and help you select which protein sources are "superfoods" for YOUR gut. It will also tell you which proteins to minimize and avoid.

If you're a vegetarian or vegan, then plant-based protein powders (such as Protein Breakthrough) are a good option.

6 Key Factors for Selecting Your Protein Powder

1 - First and foremost, you want your protein coming from whole foods. We suggest avoiding synthesized, chemically extracted protein isolates (like whey). This is critical.

2 - You want a protein that contains all the essential amino acids. In other words, it has the eight essential amino acids that your body doesn't manufacture, and it's even better if it has the other 12 that your body does make.

3 - You also want to make sure that the protein contains essential fatty acids. It helps with hormonal profile and makes for more balanced nutrition.

4 - Fiber is a critical component to your protein source, because it allows you to maintain digestive health, and slows the release of protein into the bloodstream. This is important for maintaining blood sugar. When it comes to protein, you want some fiber with it. This helps optimize bowel movements.

5 - Ideally, use A plant-based protein that's certified organic.

6 - Choose a protein that only uses natural and low-glycemic sweeteners. It's quite common for products to have artificial sweeteners, like sucralose, or aspartame. Many of these chemical

129 Micha, R., Wallace, S. K., & Mozaffarian, D. (2010). Red and processed meat consumption and risk of incident coronary heart disease, stroke, and diabetes mellitus: a systematic review and meta-analysis. *Circulation, 121*(21), 2271–2283. https://doi.org/10.1161/CIRCULATIONAHA.109.924977

130 Larsson, S. C., Bergkvist, L., & Wolk, A. (2006). Processed meat consumption, dietary nitrosamines and stomach cancer risk in a cohort of Swedish women. *International journal of cancer, 119*(4), 915–919. https://doi.org/10.1002/ijc.21925

131 Santarelli, R. L., Pierre, F., & Corpet, D. E. (2008). Processed meat and colorectal cancer: a review of epidemiologic and experimental evidence. *Nutrition and cancer, 60*(2), 131–144. https://doi.org/10.1080/01635580701684872

sweeteners negatively affect the digestive system by impacting the flora in the intestinal tract. The other issue is that it can create insulin resistance especially when consumed with carbohydrates.[132]

When it comes to sweeteners, you want to have something that's easily assimilable and recognized by the body.

That's why we use naturally grown sweeteners like monk fruit, erythritol (from birch trees), and stevia. These sweeteners are very easily assimilable. They don't cause massive spikes in blood sugar. That means over the long run we're able to stabilize blood sugar, which is essential to long-term health, weight management, and performance.

What Are the Best Fats for YOUR Body?

Genetics is possibly the most important factor in selecting which fats are the best for your body.

Generic statements like, "*coconut oil is the best fat*" and "*Saturated fats are evil*" are ignorant, uneducated opinions.

For example, some people don't have the genetics to consume, convert, and assimilate coconut oil. Matt is one of these people. He was consuming a lot of coconut oil and his triglycerides were through the roof. After cutting it out, it went back down to normal.

Some people have genes such as:

ADRB2: Plays a role in energy balance and metabolism. It's considered a "thrifty gene" because it can make our bodies more efficient, using as few calories as possible to function. While efficiency might sound good, in practical terms it means that it's easier to get more out of the calories you eat, and those extra calories are stored in our fat tissue. The GG variant is the most efficient, so those who have this may consider keeping to a l, and especially lower saturated fat, plan. The AA and AG variants are better at burning excess calories.

APOA2: The "Eat fat, get fat" gene (satiation gene). This enzyme regulates appetite. Those with the CC variant tend to have a higher BMI when saturated fats are included in the diet. The other two variants, CT and TT, do not show this association and can tolerate higher amounts of saturated fats in their diets. People who eat more fat tend to be more hungry and tend to consume more calories in a day. If you have this variation and eat a lot of fat - YOU HAVE TO MOVE and burn calories, or you will get FAT.

---

[132] Dalenberg, J. R., Patel, B. P., Denis, R., Veldhuizen, M. G., Nakamura, Y., Vinke, P. C., Luquet, S., & Small, D. M. (2020). Short-Term Consumption of Sucralose with, but Not without, Carbohydrate Impairs Neural and Metabolic Sensitivity to Sugar in Humans. *Cell metabolism, 31*(3), 493–502.e7. https://doi.org/10.1016/j.cmet.2020.01.014

FTO3: The Hangry Gene, has to do with the hunger hormone ghrelin. The FTO gene impacts on overall body fat depending on how much fat you eat, especially saturated fat. Both the CC and CT variants of this gene tend to hold on to fat more, and so you need less of it in the diet to compensate. The TT variant has an easier time of letting go of fat stores than other variants. People who have this, especially homozygous, are the people that are just hungry all the time. Balancing blood sugar is the key.

LPL: This gene helps to modulate whether saturated fats are stored as body fat or burned as fuel, and plays a role in how saturated fats are broken down for energy. Those with the GG variant of this gene break down saturated fats and use them for energy easily. However, the CG and CC variants of this gene have less ability to tolerate saturated fats in the diet, since they can be easily converted into cholesterol.

APOC3: This gene is important in regulating blood triglyceride levels as well as LDL cholesterol, which is the more dangerous type. Saturated fats in the diet are the modulating factor of how strongly a role this gene plays. Those with the CC variant of this gene have a significantly increased risk of atherosclerosis and elevated blood lipid levels when saturated fats are present in the diet. Those with the GG and GC variants do not share this increased risk.

Regardless of genetics, EFAs known as "essential fatty acids" are the most important type of fats you should focus on consuming.

Here are the top 8 best sources of EFA:

1 - Caviar (fish eggs) are the champ coming in at 6,786 mg of EFAs per 100 grams.
2 - Mackerel comes in at over 5,134 mg of EFAs per 100 grams.
3 - Herring has 2,366 mg of EFAs per 100 grams.
4 - Salmon has 2,260 mg of EFAs per 100 grams.
5 - Cod Liver oil has 2,682 mg per TBSP.
6 - Anchovies have 2,113 mg of EFAs per 100 grams.
7 - Sardines have 1,480 mg of EFAs per 100 grams.
8 - Oysters have 435 mg of EFAs per 100 grams.

Here are the top EFA options for vegetarians and vegans:

1 - Algal oil (derived from algae) has 500 mg of EFAs per dose.
2 - Perilla oil (derived from perilla seeds) has 9,000 mg of ALA omega 3 per TBSP.
3 - Flaxseeds have an epic 6,388 mg of ALA Omega 3s per ounce.
4 - Hemp seeds have a whopping 6,000 mg of ALA Omega 3s per ounce.
5 - Chia seeds have a 4,915 mg of ALA Omega 3s per ounce.
6 - Brussels sprouts come in at over 125 mg of EFAs per half cup.
7 - Walnuts have 2,542 mg of ALA Omega 3s per ounce.

Vegetarians and vegans need to have more vigilance when it comes to EFAs to make sure they're getting enough DHA. DHA is critical for brain function, eyes, reproductive function, and much more. Yes, the body can convert some of the ALA from seeds into DHA and EPA, but not efficiently. A much better source is to consume microalgae.

Fats Everyone Should Avoid

Choosing the right fats to consume is critical. However, selecting which fats to avoid is far simpler and just as important.

1 - Artificial trans fats are most likely the unhealthiest fat you can possibly eat. Be aware that on labels it's often listed as "partially hydrogenated oils". [133] [134] [135]

2 - Vegetable and most seed oils are too high in omega 6s. This imbalance in omegas can lead to inflammation. We strongly suggest avoiding or minimizing these popular cooking oil options:

- Soybean oil
- Corn oil
- Cottonseed oil
- Sunflower oil
- Peanut oil
- Sesame oil
- Rice bran oil

Micro-Nutrification: Vitamins and Minerals

Most people are familiar with the macrominerals: calcium, phosphorus, magnesium, sodium, potassium, chloride, and sulfur.

However, the body has 102 minerals that it needs to function at its peak. It's critical to give your body the right amount of trace minerals your cells need to be biologically optimized.

One easy dietary change is to upgrade your salts. Pink Himalayan salt has 84 minerals. Sea salt can have up to 75 minerals.

Is salt the enemy? Absolutely not. High-quality salt is one of the most precious things you can consume.

[133] Lopez-Garcia, E., Schulze, M. B., Meigs, J. B., Manson, J. E., Rifai, N., Stampfer, M. J., Willett, W. C., & Hu, F. B. (2005). Consumption of trans fatty acids is related to plasma biomarkers of inflammation and endothelial dysfunction. *The Journal of nutrition, 135*(3), 562–566. https://doi.org/10.1093/jn/135.3.562

[134] Calder P. C. (2015). Functional Roles of Fatty Acids and Their Effects on Human Health. JPEN. *Journal of parenteral and enteral nutrition, 39*(1 Suppl), 18S–32S. https://doi.org/10.1177/0148607115595980

[135] Kiage, J. N., Merrill, P. D., Robinson, C. J., Cao, Y., Malik, T. A., Hundley, B. C., Lao, P., Judd, S. E., Cushman, M., Howard, V. J., & Kabagambe, E. K. (2013). Intake of trans fat and all-cause mortality in the Reasons for Geographical and Racial Differences in Stroke (REGARDS) cohort. *The American journal of clinical nutrition, 97*(5), 1121–1128. https://doi.org/10.3945/ajcn.112.049064

Doesn't salt increase blood pressure and lead to more heart attacks? Let's take a look at the data from Japan.[136] [137] [138] Their heart attack rates are half of the USA.

Does sodium increase blood pressure? Yes, it does. However, there are much healthier ways to lower blood pressure. By lowering your body's overall carb levels, your blood fluid volume will drop along with your blood pressure. Lowering body fat is another effective way to lower blood pressure. Of course, consult your doctor before making these important decisions.

How to Avoid Wasting Your Money on Ground Up Rocks

According to the Dr. Reference Guide On Supplements, only 3% to 5% of a multivitamin pill is absorbed by the body.

Most multivitamins are chemicalized, unnatural vitamins and minerals that are compressed together into a pill.

They do very little good to your body if they aren't absorbed or aren't bio-available to your cells. In fact, it can be dangerous as they accumulate in the bloodstream. This happened to Matt a long time ago. He had toxic levels of vitamin Bs in his blood because he was consuming a cheap multi-vitamin that wasn't being assimilated.

When it comes to vitamins and minerals, they need to come from organic mineral deposits like humic shale, or from live plants.

Fulvic acid serves as nature's delivery system for delivering nutrients into the cell where you need them.

We want to make sure that the fulvic acid comes from a natural source and doesn't use chemical extraction.

Delivery of the nutrients is everything, so we want to have a liquid mineral and vitamin. This allows for easy absorption and assimilation, even in a person that has a compromised digestive system.

When it comes to vitamins, you want to make sure that you have a vitamin supplement that's focused on B and D vitamins, because those are the biggest sources of deficiency.

Vitamin B is vital for energy production in the body.

---

[136] Miura, K., Okuda, N., Turin, T. C., Takashima, N., Nakagawa, H., Nakamura, K., Yoshita, K., Okayama, A., Ueshima, H., & NIPPON DATA80/90 Research Group (2010). Dietary salt intake and blood pressure in a representative Japanese population: baseline analyses of NIPPON DATA80. *Journal of epidemiology, 20 Suppl 3*(Suppl 3), S524–S530. https://doi.org/10.2188/jea.je20090220

[137] *Sodium in Your Diet.* U.S. Food and Drug Administration. Retrieved 2 October 2020, from https://www.fda.gov/food/nutrition-education-resources-materials/sodium-your-diet.

[138] *CORONARY HEART DISEASE DEATH RATE BY COUNTRY.* World Life Expectancy. (2018). Retrieved 2 October 2020, from https://www.worldlifeexpectancy.com/cause-of-death/coronary-heart-disease/by-country/.

Vitamin D regulates hormone function. Having an optimal hormonal state is key in light of the toxic world that we're facing.

As far as to trace minerals, your cells function at their best when they have all 85 minerals at optimal levels. They are like the little instruments in the orchestra. Together they have a powerful effect.

As far as major minerals, magnesium is the most important and probably the most systemically deficient. Stress causes the body to excrete more magnesium. The lower the magnesium gets, the more the body shifts into a fight-flight-or-freeze response. This in turn burns more magnesium. It's a vicious cycle that most people are trapped in. This is why we recommend consuming up to 5 grams of magnesium a day spread out throughout the day as a loading phase.

Once you feel your body shift into a parasympathetic response, which you'll know because you'll feel relaxed all the time, you can lower the dose to 1 2 grams a day depending on your lifestyle.

Finally, you want to make sure you have all of the platinum group metals. Trace amounts of platinum group elements enhance cell-to-cell communication. We're often deficient in them because modern medicine focuses on major minerals like calcium.

Platinum-group minerals like gold and silver stimulate the form and function of the glands inside the body. When your glands are producing the right hormones to regulate metabolism, you have more energy and have a better ability to build the optimum biological environment that supports the growth of new cells.

When you combine everything together: enzymes, probiotics, proteins, essential fatty acids, bioavailable vitamins, and conductive minerals, you get a synergistic symphony that you can literally feel.

You'll find your energy levels sky-rocket, unhealthy food cravings diminish, and brain function and concentration levels sharpen dramatically.

Chapter 9

Biological Optimizer #1:
Nutrification, BiOptimizing Conversion of Food Into Nutrients

In this chapter, you will learn:

- **The 5 stages of digestion and how to avoid critical problems in each one.**

- Why indigestion can lead to excess inches and even sluggish metabolism.

- **The little-known nutrient that makes cheat days more enjoyable.**

- And much more...

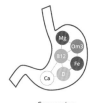

Conversion

Troubleshooting Your Digestion

Here are some questions you can answer to help you assess your digestive health:

1 - After a meal, do you feel bloated?
2 - Do you burp a lot?
3 - Do you fart a lot? Does it stink deep?
4 - How many bowel movements a day do you have? It should match the number of meals you have.
5 - Do you feel "full" for a long time after a meal?
6 - Does your stomach get upset easily?
7 - Do you ever get constipated?
8 - Do you ever get abdominal cramps?
9 - Are your stools poorly formed?
10 - Do you ever experience diarrhea?
11 - Do your stools have a pungent stench?
12 - Do you get tired after you eat?

If you answered "yes" to any of these questions, then there's room for optimizing your digestion and the answers are found in this chapter.

Optimizing The 5 Stages of Digestion

Conversion, which is converting food into usable nutrients for the body, is one of the biggest factors in determining whether or not you get value from the nutrients from food you consume. You can eat the most nutrient-rich fruits, vegetables, and meat in the world but unless it gets broken down and passes through your small intestine into your bloodstream, it's a waste of your hard-earned money.

There are 5 stages of digestion:

1 - Preparation
1 - Secretion
1 - Breakdown
1 - Absorption
1 - Elimination

Let's walk through how to optimize the 5 stages of digestion.

Stage 1: Preparation

The very first part of the digestive process begins in your mouth. Chewing tells your brain what kind of food you're eating. Then your body will begin producing the right kind of enzymes for that food.

If it's carbohydrates, it will produce amylase in your saliva. If it's protein, the submandibular glands located under your jawbone, secrete protease to help with protein breakdown. If it's fats, the sublingual glands (which means "under the tongue") help produce lipase, which aids in fat digestion.

The optimal number of chews is between 25-50 chews. However, in today's hyper-distracted world we have a chronic under-chewing epidemic. We watch TVs, social media, and rush while we eat. We strongly advise mindfully eating your food and turning off the distractions. [139] [140]

Stage 2: Secretion

After 30 minutes, hydrochloric acid and enzymes are released by the stomach. The enzymes begin the nutrient breakdown. We will go into greater depth in Stage 3.

 ## Powermove: Take the Right Enzymes for Each Meal

One of the ways to optimize your digestion is to consume the right enzymes for the meal that you're eating. A high-quality enzyme will survive the stomach acids and start breaking

[139] Accarino, A. M., Azpiroz, F., & Malagelada, J. R. (1997). Attention and distraction: effects on gut perception. *Gastroenterology, 113*(2), 415–422. https://doi.org/10.1053/gast.1997.v113.pm9247458

[140] Mason, A. E., Epel, E. S., Kristeller, J., Moran, P. J., Dallman, M., Lustig, R. H., Acree, M., Bacchetti, P., Laraia, B. A., Hecht, F. M., & Daubenmier, J. (2016). Effects of a mindfulness-based intervention on mindful eating, sweets consumption, and fasting glucose levels in obese adults: data from the SHINE randomized controlled trial. *Journal of behavioral medicine, 39*(2), 201–213. https://doi.org/10.1007/s10865-015-9692-8

down food into utilizable nutrients.

For most diets, we recommend taking MassZymes with each meal. For those who follow a ketogenic diet, we suggest taking kApex. For those times when you want to indulge, we recommend Gluten Guardian.

As food enters your stomach through a muscular ring, which opens and closes in order to keep acid from coming up into your esophagus, gastric acid (known as HCL or hydrochloric acid) and enzyme secretion become activated.

Hydrochloric acid (or HCL) helps your body to break down, digest, and absorb nutrients such as protein. It also eliminates bacteria, parasites, and viruses in the stomach, protecting your body from infection.

The Hydrochloric Acid Problem

Stomach acid, also referred to as gastric acid, is essential for the digestive process.

When the stomach cannot produce enough acid, key minerals and proteins can't be absorbed into the body. Low stomach acid is medically referred to as hypochlorhydria. It's also the primary cause of heartburn, as I'll explain in a moment.

If the body doesn't receive the necessary nutrients, you can become vitamin or mineral deficient.

Low HCL levels can leave the body vulnerable to a number of diseases and health complications, and common symptoms include:

- Upset stomach
- Nausea
- Acid reflux
- Heartburn
- Malnutrition
- Skin issues
- Osteoporosis
- Leaky gut syndrome
- Diabetes
- Cancer
- Asthma
- Rheumatoid arthritis
- Small intestinal bacterial overgrowth (SIBO)

Most people believe that heartburn and acid reflux-related issues are caused by having too much acid. It's the opposite: heartburn is caused by having too little stomach acid.

Dr. Wright, a holistic health practitioner from Lake Tahoe, has helped thousands of patients suffering from heartburn.

He says that 90% of people who visited him for heartburn were never tested for stomach acid levels, misdiagnosed, and wrongfully prescribed PPIs and antacids.

Without the proper test, patients suffering from heartburn are often assumed to have too much stomach acid and are wrongfully prescribed potentially dangerous drugs.

But the scientific literature says that heartburn and GERD (Gastroesophageal reflux disease, a.k.a. acid reflux) are not considered to be diseases of excess stomach acid.

Experts now know that acid reflux is caused by excess gas forcing the lower esophageal valve (LES) to open and allows acid to hit your throat.

Your esophageal valve is like a water dam. When you have too much gas inside your body, it "breaks the dam" and forces a "flood" of acid up your throat causing pain and discomfort in your chest. That's when you taste that bitter bile.

Yes, heartburn happens when the pressure and gas in your abdominal cavity get too high.
The main cause of excess gas is low stomach acid.

Research has proven that low stomach acid leads to both poor digestion of carbohydrates and bacterial overgrowth which causes an overload of gas.

Bad bacteria start to party and feast on poorly digested carbohydrates, especially refined carbs: sugary snacks, pizza, bread, cookies, cakes, etc.

The result is intense fermentation... and too much GAS.

Dr. Robillard's book "Heartburn Cured" reveals a shocking fact:

"30 g of carbohydrate that escapes absorption in a day could produce more than 10,000 mL of hydrogen gas. That is a huge amount of gas!"

The excess gas problem explains why PPI's and antacids often amplify acid reflux. By suppressing stomach acid with a PPI, the carb digestion becomes worse. This increases bad bacteria and fermentation even more.

In one study, 30 people with acid reflux were given 40g of Prilosec (a PPI) for at least 3 months. 11 out of the 30 developed significant bacterial overgrowth, versus 1 in 10 of people in the control group.

In Dr. Jonathan Wright's book "Why Stomach Acid Is Good For You" he tells a story of the gray man.

This man was in his 60's and his wife had brought him into Dr. Wright's holistic clinic. She was afraid that her husband's 30 years of PPI use was leading to serious health problems.
Dr. Wright had never seen anything like it.

The man's skin was gray, devoid of any pink hues. He had suffered from chronic fatigue for years.

He was originally prescribed Tagamet (an acid blocker) for his chronic heartburn and indigestion and had been taking it since it came out in 1977.

Dr. Wright asked the gray man if his doctor measured his stomach acid levels before prescribing any medication. He hadn't.

So Dr. Wright performed a simple test that measured his stomach levels. And not to Wright's surprise, the gray man's stomach acid was very low. Then Dr. Wright gave him a couple of diet changes.

He told him to slowly wean off his acid-blocking prescription medication and recommended 3 supplements: digestive enzymes, probiotics, and betaine HCl (hydrochloric acid).

The enzymes were to help break down the food in his stomach (because with age we naturally lose our ability to produce more enzymes).

The probiotics were to fight off the bad bacteria in his stomach and intestines.

The betaine HCL was the most important of all 3. It helped restore the gray man's stomach acid levels back to normal and have a healthy functioning stomach.

Dr. Wright explains:

"Slowly but surely, his gray skin color returned to normal, healthy-looking brown and pink skin tones. His fatigue dissipated, too, replaced by increasing energy. His wife also noted an improvement in his mood and attitude. Six months later, he declared himself back to normal."

In his book, Dr. Wright goes on to say: *"Even in severe cases diagnosed with acid reflux, actual testing shows hypochlorhydria in over 90 percent of cases."*

So what is betaine HCL? Betaine hydrochloride is an acidic form of betaine, a vitamin-like substance found in grains and other foods.

While I've covered carbohydrates and why HCL is so important for their digestion, it's just as important to mention protein. Those who consume animal protein REALLY need additional hydrochloric acid. That's why we suggest consuming HCL Breakthrough with each meal.

Protein is the only nutrient that needs to be prepared by hydrochloric acid before your stomach's naturally occurring enzymes can work properly.

Powermove: Consume HCL With Each Meal

If you're in your 30's or older, it might be time to consider adding HCL to your digestive stack. Adding 1 or 2 capsules of HCL Breakthrough to each meal can make a night-and-day difference to your digestion. It stacks wonderfully with enzymes and probiotics to create the ultimate digestive trio.

Here's a quick self-test for low HCl/ hypochlorhydria:

You can determine if you need HCl by a simple home test, called the bicarb test.

Instructions:

Mix 1/4 teaspoon of bicarbonate of soda (baking soda) in water (about 6 ounces) and drink on an empty stomach, first thing in the morning, before eating or drinking. If you have sufficient levels of stomach acid, the bicarbonate will be converted into carbon dioxide gas, which should cause belching within less than 5 minutes. If you have not belched within 5 minutes, stop timing.

If you have enough stomach acid, belching should occur within 2 - 3 minutes. Early and repeated belches might be due to excessive stomach acid, but they also could be due to swallowing air when drinking the solution (this sort of belching tends to be smaller belches). If 'normal' belching doesn't occur until after 3 minutes, stomach acid is low.

To recap:

Low stomach acid   —›   no belching
Sufficient stomach acid   —›   belching

The 3rd digestive substance your body produces is bile. Bile is critical for breaking down fats. It also helps us absorb fat-soluble vitamins like A, D, E, and K.

Bile is a greenish-brown fluid that helps digest fats from our food intake. It is produced by the liver and stored and concentrated in the gallbladder until it is needed to help digest foods. When food enters the small intestine, bile travels through the common bile duct to reach the duodenum.

One of the natural herbs you can take to stimulate bile production is dandelion roots, which is why we have included it inside of kApex.

Stage 3: Breakdown

Next is when we deconstruct the food into its raw elements. We break down fats into fatty acids, proteins into amino acids, and carbohydrates into glycogen.

This is where enzymes do their magic. According to Dr. Howell, the enzyme pool of an individual determines how quickly, or how well you're able to break down and absorb the nutrients you're consuming.

In today's world, we're eating a lot of cooked, processed, chemical-laden, and genetically modified foods.

Cooking Kills

Humans are the only animal that cooks its food. Cooking removes a lot of the enzymes present that would normally assist with digestion.

Remember all the food that's cooked, pasteurized, or processed with heat, does not possess any enzymes. That's why we always suggest taking a few capsules of enzymes and probiotics with every meal.

With age, our enzyme reserves get lower and lower. We absorb fewer and fewer nutrients. This leads to other problems. It's a vicious cycle.

How to Select the Right Enzymes for You

With enzymes, we're looking specifically for a full-spectrum enzyme formula that has high levels of protease designed for the full pH range of the intestinal tract. This is because different amino acids are assimilated at different pH levels.

That's why we created a tri-phase protease formulation that contains not just one protease, but three different proteases in our medical-grade enzyme formula: MassZymes.
These proteases work at various pHs so that we get maximum assimilation of amino acids.

It's a critical point of digestion because if you miss the pH window of digestion, certain amino acids don't get broken down. As we learned in INSERT CHAPTER, amino acids are crucial for our health. Most enzyme formulations are low on protease simply because it's very expensive to produce.

You also want an enzymatic formulation that is stable, utilizable, and based on a plant-based formulation as opposed to an animal-based.

A lot of companies go to animal-based enzymes because they're less expensive. We've found that animal-based enzymes don't work nearly as well as plant-based enzymes. Animal enzymes tend to be less consistent in strength and function.

Also, it's good to have a multipurpose enzyme containing the other enzymes, such as lactase, amylase, lipase, and other enzymes. Each enzyme breaks down specific macronutrients. For example, amylase digests carbohydrates and sugars. Lipase breaks down fats into usable fatty acids.

We suggest taking 2 to 5 capsules of a high-quality enzyme formulation with every meal, especially when you eat flesh protein such as fish or meat, to maximize the amino acid absorption.

Stage 4: Absorption

Your digestive system is a tube that's up to 30 feet long from your mouth to your anus. These valuable nutrients you're consuming have zero benefits for you unless they pass from that tube into your bloodstream. That's what the absorption stage is all about.

As food enters the small intestine, the process shifts to absorption — and this is where your microbiome plays a critical role. Friendly microbes in your gut can actually further stimulate enzymes to help break down any food that wasn't fully processed earlier.

This is why consuming foods high in probiotics can aid in digestion.

Here are the richest foods in probiotics:

1 - Real Yogurt: Most of the commercial yogurts are filled with dead probiotics and an overload of sugar. Real yogurt is incredibly sour to the taste because the live probiotics have consumed the sugar and produced beneficial acids.

2 - Kefir: Closely resembles that of yogurt. It will provide a good dose of calcium as well as healthy bacteria. Try and choose kefir that is unflavored or the added sugar found in it may help to prevent the healthy bacteria from thriving inside the body.

3 - Sauerkraut: The primary bacteria found in this type of food is Lactobacillus, which is found in concentrations even higher than that of yogurt. Prepare sauerkraut yourself rather than purchase a store variety because they are typically prepared using vinegar, which kills off much of the beneficial bacteria.

4 - Tempeh: Tempeh not only provides a good dose of protein, but is also an excellent way to boost your probiotic intake, and it's a great source of calcium.

5 - Kimchi: Kimchi is prepared using cabbage, radishes, scallions and may also contain red pepper or salted shrimp. The probiotic strain found in kimchi is called Lactobacillus Brevis and may help promote greater weight loss.

6 - Miso: Miso soup is made from fermented soybeans along with salt and koji, which is a fungus that's edible. Taking miso in helps to boost your digestive system, enhance your immune system, and may also help to lower your overall risk factor for cancer as well.[141] [142]

7 - Kombucha: Kombucha is one of the fermented probiotic drinks that is made with black or green tea along with yeast that helps to ferment it.

8 - Pickles: You want to get fermented pickles, which are usually best made yourself. You don't need any ingredients besides cucumbers (or any other vegetable you desire), salt, and water. The good news is if you choose to make your own, you can sidestep many of the additives that are included with the ones that you purchase off the supermarket shelves.

9 - Natto: Natto is a Japanese dish that is basically made from fermented soybeans and has a sticky sort of texture. This dish is very rich in vitamin K and has been known to help boost skin health as well, preventing wrinkles and boosting skin elasticity.[143]

10 - Raw fruits and vegetables: Are a great natural source of probiotics and have a very diverse range of live bacteria.

Research has shown that bacteria will help nutrient absorption — from macronutrients like protein and fats to micronutrients. Human studies have shown that higher levels of prebiotics, probiotics, and synbiotics (food that creates synergy with the probiotics, they're usually high in fiber and prebiotics) in the diet increase mineral absorption, bone mineral content, and bone structure.

We also recommend taking probiotics with your meal for maximum digestion -- Their role is not only to colonize the gut but rather to assist in the digestion and absorption process. Their other role is to "clean house" and help eliminate bad bacteria.

Wade and Matt talked with Naveen Jain about the data he's seen with Viome's gut tests. He said, he almost never sees any commercial probiotics inside stool samples. Our native probiotic levels are determined more by what we eat (and what we avoid) than the probiotic supplements we take.

The best plan of action is to eat a variety of foods, especially vegetables for microbial diversity, and combine that with a probiotic-based on how well it helps you breakdown your food.

---

[141] Clemente, J. C., Ursell, L. K., Parfrey, L. W., & Knight, R. (2012). The impact of the gut microbiota on human health: an integrative view. *Cell, 148*(6), 1258–1270. https://doi.org/10.1016/j.cell.2012.01.035

[142] Brown, A. C., & Valiere, A. (2004). Probiotics and medical nutrition therapy. *Nutrition in clinical care : an official publication of Tufts University, 7*(2), 56–68.

[143] Hsu, M. F., & Chiang, B. H. (2009). Stimulating effects of Bacillus subtilis natto-fermented Radix astragali on hyaluronic acid production in human skin cells. *Journal of ethnopharmacology, 125*(3), 474–481. https://doi.org/10.1016/j.jep.2009.07.011

The Probiotic Protocol

In regards to probiotics, there are a couple of key components. You want to have a bacteria strain that is transient.

You want powerful bacteria that can overthrow bad bacteria. In other words, a strain that's strong enough to wipe-out bacteria cultures that have been taken over your digestive terrain.

Here's a big key: you want a potent proteolytic probiotic strain. This means the probiotic will help you digest protein.

Stage 5: Elimination

After all that hard work, it's time to ship out the waste to the great sewer in the ground!

Whatever's left at this point, enters the colon. Most of the water will be reabsorbed by the body. This is one of the reasons why consuming water-rich fruits and veggies can help digestion.

Probiotics continue to play a role in the colon, continuing the breakdown process. Peristaltic movements continue to help move the semi-solid waste through the colon.

At this stage, your rectum expands in response to the storage of fecal matter. Using peristaltic movements of the rectum, waste is ultimately eliminated through the anus, completing the digestive process.

The success of this process often has a lot to do with the stages before it. Otherwise, without adequate enzymes, hydrochloric acid, and digestion-enhancing probiotics, undigested food will make it to the colon.

Probiotics, Enzymes, and HCL:
The Ultimate 1-2-3 Trio That Solves 99% of Digestive Issues

With our 50,000 customers, the following digestive stack has solved virtually every single person's problems and moved them much further down the BiOptimization Spectrum towards super-human health.

1 - HCL Breakthrough
2 - MassZymes
3 - P3OM

These help optimize all 5 of the digestive stages. HCL Breakthrough has a powerful impact on the first stage. It helps break down the food and prepare it for the digestive stage.

MassZymes is the ultimate enzyme formula. Its proteolytic enzymes convert the proteins into amino acids. P3OM also aids in breaking down the protein into amino acids. The Astrazyme helps transport those amino acids into the bloodstream.

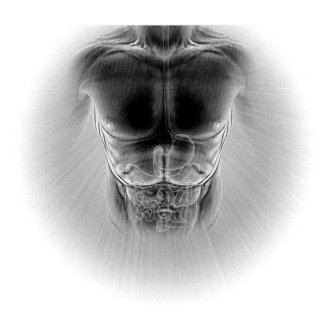

P3OM then continues to do its magic in the final stages to maximize the value you're getting from the food you consume.

Your body can then use those amino acids to produce neurotransmitters (which are vital to the health of your brain). Your body will also use amino acids to rebuild muscle tissue. They are vital to speed up the recovery from your workouts.

HCL, probiotics, and enzymes will help you ASSIMILATE maximum nutrients from the food you eat. They are the foundation of your BiOptimization Blueprint.

Transporting Amino Acids Through the Intestinal Tract

As noted above, we've added a special ingredient called Astrazymes to MassZymes to improve its effectiveness even more. It's an astragalus based ingredient that helps transport up to 70% more amino acids through the intestinal tract. That's the key to maximize the absorption phase.

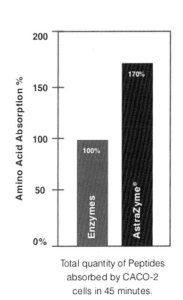

Total quantity of Peptides absorbed by CACO-2 cells in 45 minutes.

Chapter 10

Biological Optimizer #1: Nutrification, BiOptimizing Assimilation

In this chapter, you will learn:

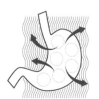
Assimilation

- **The TRUTH about glucose and how to know if you're getting enough or too little.**

- How to double the breakdown of the fats you eat.

- **The 1 nutrient you MUST have to turn protein into muscle.**

- And much more...

Now the nutrients have entered your bloodstream. Technically, you're not nutrified until the nutrients become assimilated in your body.

How Does the Body Assimilate Glucose?

Simply stated: it either becomes utilized for energy or it gets stored.

More specifically it does one of 4 things:

1 - Become burned for energy by synthesizing adenosine triphosphate (ATP).
2 - Become stored in the liver.
3 - Become stored in the muscle tissue.
4 - Becomes body fat via gluconeogenesis.

One of the keys to avoiding health problems and minimizing body fat gain is keeping a high level of insulin sensitivity.

Monitoring your blood sugar is one of the best ways to BiOptimize this. If your fasted blood sugar creeps up too much, you should start taking steps to lower this. Ideally, your fasted blood sugar is between 80-94. 100 to 125 is considered suboptimal. If it's 126 on two different tests, you have diabetes.

Some simple tips to manage blood sugar and insulin resistance:

1 - Take a 10 min walk after each meal.[144] [145] Credit goes to Stan Efferding for bringing awareness to this simple, powerful tip.

---

[144] Reynolds, A. N., Mann, J. I., Williams, S., & Venn, B. J. (2016). Advice to walk after meals is more effective for lowering postprandial glycaemia in type 2 diabetes mellitus than advice that does not specify timing: a randomised crossover study. *Diabetologia, 59*(12), 2572–2578. https://doi.org/10.1007/s00125-016-4085-2

[145] Smith, A. D., Crippa, A., Woodcock, J., & Brage, S. (2016). Physical activity and incident type 2 diabetes mellitus: a systematic review and dose-response meta-analysis of prospective cohort studies. *Diabetologia, 59*(12), 2527–2545. https://doi.org/10.1007/s00125-016-4079-0

---

2 - Get great sleep.[146] [147] [148] [149] [150]

3 - Eat lower glycemic carbs.

4 - Lower daily carb intake.

5 - If extreme measures need to be taken, eliminate carbs entirely for a few weeks.[151] [152]

6 - Add magnesium to your supplement stack.[153] [154]

7 - Add spices to your diet: specifically curcumin,[155] ginger,[156] garlic,[157] ceylon, cinnamon, and fenugreek.[158]

[146] González-Ortiz, M., Martínez-Abundis, E., Balcázar-Muñoz, B. R., & Pascoe-González, S. (2000). Effect of sleep deprivation on insulin sensitivity and cortisol concentration in healthy subjects. *Diabetes, nutrition & metabolism, 13*(2), 80–83.
[147] Donga, E., van Dijk, M., van Dijk, J. G., Biermasz, N. R., Lammers, G. J., van Kralingen, K. W., Corssmit, E. P., & Romijn, J. A. (2010). A single night of partial sleep deprivation induces insulin resistance in multiple metabolic pathways in healthy subjects. *The Journal of clinical endocrinology and metabolism, 95*(6), 2963–2968. https://doi.org/10.1210/jc.2009-2430
[148] Borghouts, L. B., & Keizer, H. A. (2000). Exercise and insulin sensitivity: a review. *International journal of sports medicine, 21*(1), 1–12. https://doi.org/10.1055/s-2000-8847
[149] Way, K. L., Hackett, D. A., Baker, M. K., & Johnson, N. A. (2016). The Effect of Regular Exercise on Insulin Sensitivity in Type 2 Diabetes Mellitus: A Systematic Review and Meta-Analysis. *Diabetes & metabolism journal, 40*(4), 253–271. https://doi.org/10.4093/dmj.2016.40.4.253
[150] Ishii, T., Yamakita, T., Sato, T., Tanaka, S., & Fujii, S. (1998). Resistance training improves insulin sensitivity in NIDDM subjects without altering maximal oxygen uptake. *Diabetes care, 21*(8), 1353–1355. https://doi.org/10.2337/diacare.21.8.1353
[151] Holmäng, A., & Björntorp, P. (1992). The effects of cortisol on insulin sensitivity in muscle. *Acta physiologica Scandinavica, 144*(4), 425–431. https://doi.org/10.1111/j.1748-1716.1992.tb09316.x
[152] Adam, T. C., Hasson, R. E., Ventura, E. E., Toledo-Corral, C., Le, K. A., Mahurkar, S., Lane, C. J., Weigensberg, M. J., & Goran, M. I. (2010). Cortisol is negatively associated with insulin sensitivity in overweight Latino youth. *The Journal of clinical endocrinology and metabolism, 95*(10), 4729–4735. https://doi.org/10.1210/jc.2010-0322
[153] de Lordes Lima, M., Cruz, T., Pousada, J. C., Rodrigues, L. E., Barbosa, K., & Canguçu, V. (1998). The effect of magnesium supplementation in increasing doses on the control of type 2 diabetes. *Diabetes care, 21*(5), 682–686. https://doi.org/10.2337/diacare.21.5.682
[154] Morais, J., Severo, J. S., de Alencar, G., de Oliveira, A., Cruz, K., Marreiro, D., Freitas, B., de Carvalho, C., Martins, M., & Frota, K. (2017). Effect of magnesium supplementation on insulin resistance in humans: A systematic review. *Nutrition (Burbank, Los Angeles County, Calif.), 38*, 54–60. https://doi.org/10.1016/j.nut.2017.01.009
[155] Kim, T., Davis, J., Zhang, A. J., He, X., & Mathews, S. T. (2009). Curcumin activates AMPK and suppresses gluconeogenic gene expression in hepatoma cells. *Biochemical and biophysical research communications, 388*(2), 377–382. https://doi.org/10.1016/j.bbrc.2009.08.018
[156] Jalal, R., Bagheri, S. M., Moghimi, A., & Rasuli, M. B. (2007). Hypoglycemic effect of aqueous shallot and garlic extracts in rats with fructose-induced insulin resistance. *Journal of clinical biochemistry and nutrition, 41*(3), 218–223. https://doi.org/10.3164/jcbn.2007031
[157] Li, Y., Tran, V. H., Duke, C. C., & Roufogalis, B. D. (2012). Gingerols of Zingiber officinale enhance glucose uptake by increasing cell surface GLUT4 in cultured L6 myotubes. *Planta medica, 78*(14), 1549–1555. https://doi.org/10.1055/s-0032-1315041
[158] Gupta, A., Gupta, R., & Lal, B. (2001). Effect of Trigonella foenum-graecum (fenugreek) seeds on glycaemic control and insulin resistance in type 2 diabetes mellitus: a double blind placebo controlled study. *The Journal of the Association of Physicians of India, 49*, 1057–1061.

8 - Do cold therapy: cryotherapy or cold baths. If you track your blood sugar, you'll see a rapid drop in your blood sugar.[159] [160] [161]

How Does the Body Assimilate Fatty Acids?

Once fats are broken down into fatty acids and glycerol by lipase and bile, they're ready to enter the bloodstream.[162]

The liver will send the fats to the muscle cell for energy or the adipose fat cell for storage.

If they aren't utilized for energy, the fatty acids are stored in body fat. And the glycerol gets stored in the liver. Glycerol has the ability to be converted into glucose.[163] This can happen when someone has low blood glucose levels caused by fasting or low carb diet. Then the liver can release that glucose to the brain for fuel.

The fatty acid will be broken down into acetyl CoA via a process called fatty acid oxidation. Once it gets broken down, it will enter the Krebs cycle and produce ATP.

We created a very special formula to help maximize this process. It's called kApex.

From the moment you take your kApex® capsules, the formula goes to work in your body:

First, kApex® helps break down the fat you eat into usable fatty acids.

The proprietary LIP4™ blend of 4 lipases (the enzymes that break down fats) in kApex® dissolve fats into easily burnable fatty acids.

It's also why the right types and amounts of lipase—are a life-saver for people struggling with digestive issues when they eat a high-fat diet including meat, fish, or other types of fat (including healthy fats).

In a study in which people ate high-fat food, patients who supplemented with lipase enzymes experienced significant reductions in bloating, gas, and fullness compared to those taking a placebo.[164]

[159] Yin, J., Xing, H., & Ye, J. (2008). Efficacy of berberine in patients with type 2 diabetes mellitus. *Metabolism: clinical and experimental, 57*(5), 712–717. https://doi.org/10.1016/j.metabol.2008.01.013

[160] Pang, B., Zhao, L. H., Zhou, Q., Zhao, T. Y., Wang, H., Gu, C. J., & Tong, X. L. (2015). Application of berberine on treating type 2 diabetes mellitus. *International journal of endocrinology, 2015,* 905749. https://doi.org/10.1155/2015/905749

[161] Dong, H., Wang, N., Zhao, L., & Lu, F. (2012). Berberine in the treatment of type 2 diabetes mellitus: a systemic review and meta-analysis. *Evidence-based complementary and alternative medicine : eCAM, 2012,* 591654. https://doi.org/10.1155/2012/591654

[162] Griffin, B. (2013). Lipid metabolism. *Surgery (Oxford), 31*(6), 267-272. https://doi.org/10.1016/j.mpsur.2013.04.006

[163] Berg, J., Tymoczko, J., & Stryer, L. (2002). *Biochemistry.* W.H. Freeman and Co.

[164] Freddi, R., Duca, P., Gritti, I., Mariotti, M., & Vertemati, M. (2009). Behavioral and degeneration changes in the basal forebrain systems of aged rats: a quantitative study in the region of the basal forebrain after levo-acetyl-carnitine treatments assessed by Abercrombie estimation. *Progress in neuro-psychopharmacology & biological psychiatry, 33*(3), 419–426. https://doi.org/10.1016/j.pnpbp.2008.12.021

We included HCL (hydrochloric acid which is stomach acid) in kApex® to assist the lipase and protease in breaking down those macronutrients.

We also included dandelion root in order to stimulate your bile flow needed for high-fat meals... so you further maximize the breakdown of fats into usable fatty acids.[165]

Second, kApex® assists in the transport of those fatty acids to your liver and your mitochondria. The L-carnitine inside helps transport the fatty acids into your liver and muscles.

Third, by enhancing mitochondrial function —kApex® helps you burn more fatty acids at an accelerated rate.

InnoSlim® helps support fat loss in multiple ways:

- Boosts AMPK in muscles by 52% and fat cells by 300% [166]
- Ups ATP in your liver by 22% [167]
- Amps adiponectin by up to 248% (a key fat-burning hormone) [168]
- Lifts GLUT4 up to 488%—which is the insulin-regulated glucose transporter found primarily in fat and muscle tissues. [169]

Then we added 7-Keto DHEA to boost a few key liver enzymes. 7-Keto is used specifically for cell metabolism and by the brain. 7-keto and its derivatives activate PPAR alpha, which is a protein that helps make peroxisomes, burn fat, and boosts weight loss.

Finally, we added CoQ10 to boost mitochondrial function. This creates the perfect synergy for turning fats into fuel.

We suggest taking 3-5 capsules on an empty stomach in the morning for 8-12 hours of energy. And 1-2 caps per meal.

[165] Passeri, M., Iannuccelli, M., Ciotti, G., Bonati, P. A., Nolfe, G., & Cucinotta, D. (1988). Mental impairment in aging: selection of patients, methods of evaluation and therapeutic possibilities of acetyl-L-carnitine. *International journal of clinical pharmacology research, 8*(5), 367–376.
[166] Pooyandjoo, M., Nouhi, M., Shab-Bidar, S., Djafarian, K., & Olyaeemanesh, A. (2016). The effect of (L-)carnitine on weight loss in adults: a systematic review and meta-analysis of randomized controlled trials. *Obesity reviews : an official journal of the International Association for the Study of Obesity, 17*(10), 970–976. https://doi.org/10.1111/obr.12436
[167] Kraemer, W. J., Volek, J. S., French, D. N., Rubin, M. R., Sharman, M. J., Gómez, A. L., Ratamess, N. A., Newton, R. U., Jemiolo, B., Craig, B. W., & Häkkinen, K. (2003). The effects of L-carnitine L-tartrate supplementation on hormonal responses to resistance exercise and recovery. *Journal of strength and conditioning research, 17*(3), 455–462. https://doi.org/10.1519/1533-4287(2003)017<0455:teolls>2.0.co;2
[168] Volek, J. S., Kraemer, W. J., Rubin, M. R., Gómez, A. L., Ratamess, N. A., & Gaynor, P. (2002). L-Carnitine L-tartrate supplementation favorably affects markers of recovery from exercise stress. *American journal of physiology. Endocrinology and metabolism, 282*(2), E474–E482. https://doi.org/10.1152/ajpendo.00277.2001
[169] Spiering, B. A., Kraemer, W. J., Hatfield, D. L., Vingren, J. L., Fragala, M. S., Ho, J. Y., Thomas, G. A., Häkkinen, K., & Volek, J. S. (2008). Effects of L-carnitine L-tartrate supplementation on muscle oxygenation responses to resistance exercise. *Journal of strength and conditioning research, 22*(4), 1130–1135. https://doi.org/10.1519/JSC.0b013e31817d48d9

How Does the Body Assimilate Amino Acids?

Each amino acid has a different role in the human body. Upon absorption, some amino acids are incorporated to create new proteins. Some fuel your muscles and support tissue repair. Others are used as a source of energy.

Tryptophan and tyrosine, for example, promote brain health. These amino acids support the production of neurotransmitters, leading to increased alertness and optimum nerve responses. Tryptophan also assists with serotonin production, lifting your mood, and keeping depression at bay.

Phenylalanine serves as a precursor to melatonin, epinephrine, dopamine, and other chemicals that regulate your mood and bodily functions.

Methionine helps your body absorb selenium and zinc, two minerals that promote overall health.

Some amino acids, such as isoleucine, play a vital role in hemoglobin production and glucose metabolism.

The "star" of the show that makes all of these metabolic processes happen is ENZYMES. Enzymes are the main "workers" that are responsible for over 25,000 different functions in the body.

Dr. Edward Howell, in his book Enzyme Nutrition,[170] stated that we are all born with an enzymatic bank account, and the more cooked food, drugs, and stress we experience, the more we spend these enzymes. Modern processed foods and the use of glyphosates are speeding up these "expenditures".

If you take proteolytic enzymes with food, they will break the protein down into absorbable amino acids and help fill up the "amino acid bank account". If you take them on an empty stomach, they can have profound systemic effects. By "systemic", we mean affecting the whole body. The research on this is startling.

A high dose of protease taken while in a fasted state has been proven to be one of the most powerful recovery tools.

Dr. Fulgrave believes that recovery from sprains and strains can go from 8 weeks of inactivity to 2 weeks with proteolytic enzymes.[171]

J.M. Zuschlag "Double-Blind Clinical Study Using Certain Proteolytic Enzymes Mixtures In Karate Fighters" study showed startling improvements:[172] from the book Enzymes Enzyme Therapy:

[170] Howell, E., & Murray, M. (1985). *Enzyme nutrition.* Avery Pub. Group.

[171] FULLGRABE E. A. (1957). Clinical experiences with chymotrypsin. *Annals of the New York Academy of Sciences, 68*(1), 192–195. https://doi.org/10.1111/j.1749-6632.1957.tb42624.x

[172] Zuschlag JM. Double-blind clinical study using certain proteolytic enzyme mixtures in karate fighters. Working paper. Mucos Pharma GmbH (Germany). 1988;1-5.

- Hematoma: 15.6 days to 6.6 days
- Swelling: 10 days to 4 days
- Restriction of movement: 12.6 days to 5 days
- Inflammation: 10.5 days to 3.8 days
- Unfit for training: 10.2 days to 4.2 days

Proteolytic enzymes taken on an empty stomach have profound effects on inflammation.

Here are the mechanisms of action:

1 - Breaking down undigested proteins in your gut that is causing inflammation.

2 - Speeding up the elimination of inflammatory proteins via your bloodstream and lymphatic system.

3 - Some cancer doctors are using high dosage proteolytic enzymes in their therapies. The theory is that cancer cells hide under a cloak of fibrin to avoid detection. Once the cancer cells' walls are broken down by the proteolytic enzymes, they can be spotted and attacked by your immune system. Fibrin accumulation creates scar tissue in damaged muscle or at a surgical site. Sometimes the scar tissue may lead to other chronic problems. The proteases can break down this fibrin.

4 - Reducing edema in the inflamed region as seen with the karate fighters.

5 - Significantly increasing the potency of macrophages and killer cells, which can positively impact immunity.

This is why we believe in taking high doses of MassZymes on an empty stomach. We believe once they enter the bloodstream, they will assist in metabolic functions. They can help breakdown proteins in the blood, which is a major cause of aging.

Conclusion

1 - The key to maximizing your assimilation of amino acids is to consume a lot of proteolytic enzymes both with food and on an empty stomach.

2 - The key to maximizing the assimilation of fatty acids is to improve the breakdown of fats using lipase, transport the fatty acids to your liver, activate more liver enzymes, and increase mitochondrial function.

Chapter 11

Biological Optimizer #2: Sleep Deep and Dominate

In this chapter, you will learn:

High Quality Sleep

- **Why poor sleep, hormonal issues, and obesity go hand in hand.**

- The 6 most dangerous sleep disruptors and how to fix them.

- **How to hack your deep sleep and wake up rested and energized.**

- And much more...

"The root of all evil is sleep deprivation."
Christophe Clugston, poly-linguist and self-defense expert.

If you were to ask Matt, *"What's the #1 thing I can do to improve all 3 sides of the BiOptimization Triangle?"* His answer would be high-quality sleep.

Sleep Deprivation Will Destroy Your Health, Your Performance, and Your Aesthetics

In his early 20s, Matt was obsessed with being as productive as possible.

- He was working in the gym 80 hours a week
- Writing a book
- Studying marketing
- Recording a hard rock album
- Training twice a day
- Teaching and training self-defense

He thought sleep was getting in the way of life. He slowly lowered his sleep by 15 minutes every few days. After a few months, he was down to 4 hours a night. He had pushed his body to the edge.

He eventually crashed and burned after months of 80 hour work weeks, 4 hours of sleep a night, and 12 workouts a week.

Then he decided to start researching sleep. He read a book called "Power Sleep" by Dr. James Mass. His main takeaway was: sleep more.
So Matt became obsessed with sleep quantity. Matt would sleep 9 hours a night, lose 3-4 lbs of water weight and wake up feeling tired, groggy, and mentally foggy. This was the norm for over a decade.

All of this changed when he started tracking his sleep using devices like the Zeo and Oura Ring. Matt was shocked to see that he was barely getting any deep sleep. It was between zero and 15 minutes per night.

This coincided with a high body fat DEXA reading and a low testosterone blood test. This was one of those wake-up calls for Matt. He realized it's about sleep quality, not quantity.

Here's what Matt says in his own words, *"I realized that improving the quality of my sleep was the #1 thing I could do to improve every aspect of my life. By dramatically improving my sleep, I would improve my appearance, improve my brain, improve my productivity, improve my sex life, and improve my health. I realized that it was the best monetary investment I could make in myself by a long shot."*

He began doing relentless research and going crazy doing experiments. After spending over $40,000 in sleep and health gear plus diving into research and chatting with fellow biohackers, there are some critical things that move the needle.

However, before we dive into the tactical and strategic things you can do, let us blow your mind with some shocking data. I want to give credit to Dan Garner and his book "Eat, Sleep, Burn" for the collection and curation of mind-opening sleep research.

Sleep deprivation is a pandemic. Here are some key data points:

- *67% of all Americans report frequent sleep issues.*
- *43% say that these sleep issues affect their daily activities.*
- *between 9-12% of the population is clinically diagnosed with insomnia.*
- *35.3% of people reported less than 7hrs of sleep per night.*
- *38% report unintentionally falling asleep throughout the day.*
- *4.7% admitted to falling asleep while driving at least once in the past month prior to when the survey was conducted.*

The real question is, what are the consequences of bad sleep?

The short answer is, you're going to get fatter, lose muscle, destroy your willpower, be in a horrible mood and crash your immune system.[173]

The groups who consistently had less sleep have higher levels of catabolic (muscle destroying) hormones such as cortisol, and also had lower levels of anabolic (muscle building) hormones such as testosterone and IGF-1.

Research has shown that low levels of sleep (5.5hrs nightly) significantly raises your body's Respiratory Exchange Ratio (RER).

Dan Garner elaborates on the consequences of this in his book, "Eat, Sleep Burn".

---

[173] Leproult, R., & Van Cauter, E. (2011). Effect of 1 week of sleep restriction on testosterone levels in young healthy men. *JAMA, 305*(21), 2173–2174. https://doi.org/10.1001/jama.2011.710

"If you are consistently getting poor sleep you are shifting the majority of your daily calorie burn to lean tissue as opposed to fatty tissue. Ideally, we would have a low RER value to optimize fat burning while keeping your lean muscle mass.

Decreased sleep level raises your RER value without affecting your basal metabolic rate. Meaning, if your daily calorie burn average is 2,500 calories, it is going to stay that way with or without a bad sleep. So, if you get a bad sleep and your RER rises, your metabolism won't lower to offer up some damage control.

You will just lose that much more lean tissue. A high metabolism combined with a high RER means a whole lot of unnecessary muscle loss due to a factor that is totally independent of nutrition and training.

To put things into perspective and give some examples. Let's say you have an average calorie burn of 2,500 calories per day. If you have a low RER value, 2000 of that could be coming from fat and only 500 from lean tissue. Whereas if you have a high RER value, 1,250 could be coming from fat at 1,250 from lean muscle tissue. Not a good trade-off if optimizing your performance potential and body composition are in your sights.

If you're trying to lose weight, do you want to lose 50% body fat and 50% lean muscle tissue? Or would you rather lose a lot more body fat and not any lean muscle tissue? This also works in the other direction. If you're trying to gain weight and lean muscle mass but you sleep poorly on a regular basis, you're going to be spinning your tires in the mud. Going nowhere fast."

Here's what the research has discovered:

A two-week experiment was done on 10 overweight adults.[174] *The 5.5hrs of sleep per night group lost 55% less fat and 60% more muscle than 8.5hrs of sleep per night group.* Beyond this, the 5.5hrs group also reported greater cravings than the 8.5hrs group. Cravings kill diets. If you can't manage hunger and cravings, your odds of success with any diet are close to zero. Sleep deprivation can easily lead to out of control food cravings.

The problems don't end there. Here are some other eye-opening data around sleep deprivation:

- Increased their levels of the hormone ghrelin by 28% (the hunger hormone).[175]

- Short-term sleep deprivation increased energy intake and led to a net weight gain in women.[176]

- Has a harmful impact on carbohydrate metabolism and endocrine function. The effects are

---

174 Nedeltcheva, A. V., Kilkus, J. M., Imperial, J., Schoeller, D. A., & Penev, P. D. (2010). Insufficient sleep undermines dietary efforts to reduce adiposity. *Annals of internal medicine, 153*(7), 435–441. https://doi.org/10.7326/0003-4819-153-7-201010050-00006

175 Morselli, L., Leproult, R., Balbo, M., & Spiegel, K. (2010). Role of sleep duration in the regulation of glucose metabolism and appetite. Best practice & research. *Clinical endocrinology & metabolism, 24*(5), 687–702. https://doi.org/10.1016/j.beem.2010.07.005

176 Bosy-Westphal, A., Hinrichs, S., Jauch-Chara, K., Hitze, B., Later, W., Wilms, B., Settler, U., Peters, A., Kiosz, D., & Muller, M. J. (2008). Influence of partial sleep deprivation on energy balance and insulin sensitivity in healthy women. Obesity facts, 1(5), 266–273. https://doi.org/10.1159/000158874

---

similar to those seen in normal aging and, therefore, may increase the severity of age-related chronic disorders.[177]

What about your brain?

- Sleep deprivation might curtail the formation of fear memories after stressful events.[178]

- Reduces the ability to perform cognitive tasks, such as executive decision making, categorizing, spatial memory, fluid verbal expression, creativity, planning tasks, detecting changes in the environment, etc.

- Leads to a strong subjective experience of fatigue, sleepiness, and pain, and in some cases to bad moods and stress.[179]

Your emotional state is going to be in a bad place. Mood swings, anger burst, and depressiveness can easily emerge.

Your ability to focus and stay alert becomes severely compromised.

Want to crash your immune system? One bad night's sleep can crash your immune system.

We could fill an entire book with research showing the negative effects of sleep deprivation. However, that's not very helpful so let's switch gears into the solution.

Eliminate the 6 Sleep Disruptors

1 - Light
2 - Pressure points
3 - Temperature
4 - Cortisol, Adrenaline, and Noradrenaline
5 - The Full Belly
6 - Crazy Beta Brain Train

There are 6 things that disrupt the body and prevent it from getting into stage 4 sleep and getting good REM.

---

177 Spiegel, K., Leproult, R., & Van Cauter, E. (1999). Impact of sleep debt on metabolic and endocrine function. *Lancet (London, England), 354*(9188), 1435–1439. https://doi.org/10.1016/S0140-6736(99)01376-8
178 Menz, M. M., Rihm, J. S., Salari, N., Born, J., Kalisch, R., Pape, H. C., Marshall, L., & Büchel, C. (2013). The role of sleep and sleep deprivation in consolidating fear memories. *NeuroImage, 75*, 87–96. https://doi.org/10.1016/j.neuroimage.2013.03.001
179 Trošt Bobić, T., Šećić, A., Zavoreo, I., Matijević, V., Filipović, B., Kolak, Ž., Bašić Kes, V., Ciliga, D., & Sajković, D. (2016). The Impact of Sleep Deprivation on the Brain. *Acta clinica Croatica, 55*(3), 469–473. https://doi.org/10.20471/acc.2016.55.03.17

Here Are the Disruptors and Their Antidotes

Sleep BiOptimizer #1: Darkness and Light

One of the simplest health hacks you can do is to optimize the light in your life. Your circadian rhythms are primarily dictated by light.

Light

First, in the morning, the blue light hitting the photoreceptors in your skin and eyes tells your body "This is the start of the day."

And then at night, the absence of light tells your brain "It's time to go to sleep." The problem is that all of our devices are fooling our brains. There's far too much blue light coming from your smartphone, tablets, TVs, and light bulbs. The brain thinks it's still day time.

This means the body doesn't produce the optimal amount of melatonin, which is critical to kickstart the sleep cycle.

Here are some thoughts on this from neurosurgeon and health researcher, Jack Kruse:

"Humans are built to burn fat at night as we sleep to lose excess weight we don't need. The timing of the leptin action is also critical. It usually occurs between 12-2 AM and is tied to when you last ate and how much darkness your eyes have seen. This generally occurs soon after our hypothalamus releases another hormone called prolactin from our pituitary gland in the brain.

Ok, you must be asking why is this prolactin hormone so important? Is not prolactin just a hormone to secrete human milk, doc? That is not the only action of prolactin. Immediately after prolactin is released at this time, another signal is sent to the anterior pituitary to release Growth Hormone (GH). GH is stimulated only during autophagic sleep cycles in stages 3 and 4 to increase protein synthesis for muscle growth all while you're dissipating heat.

This is the major release of GH in humans post puberty. The implications here are huge. If you are leptin resistant and have sleep apnea you will have an altered body composition because of a low GH level. It means as you age you have higher body fat and lower muscle mass. This is precisely what we see in humans as they age and invariably their sleep is also poor."

There are 3 ways to use light and darkness to optimize your sleep.

1) Eliminate the blue lights before bed

Your body will NOT produce melatonin if there's too much blue light before sleep. You have a few options. At night, only turn on the orangeish bulbs such as those found here.

Your second option is to wear blue light blocking glasses. Check out the book's reference guide for our recommendations.

2) Sleep in total darkness

Your body will not produce melatonin if it's being hit by light while you're sleeping. Your bedroom should be so dark, that you can't see your hand with your eyes open. Matt has 2 layers of blackout curtains to make sure not a lumen of light comes in.

Matt wore a sleep mask for years. The problem is, your skin has photoreceptors. So your sleep will be disrupted by the light hitting your skin.

There is only one option here: create a pitch-black room. We suggest getting 2 layers of good light-absorbing shades on Amazon.

Powermove: Garbage Bags and Black Tape

Make sure to cover every electronic light in your room with black electrical tape or something similar. Even those will have an effect.

Here's a pro tip while you travel: buy heavy-duty garbage bags and tape them to the window of your room. It's a cheap, easy "hack" to eliminate unwanted light.

3) Blast your eyes with blue light in the morning

This is a highly underrated sleep hack. And this is one of the most powerful ways to reset your circadian rhythm when traveling.

By blasting your eyes with blue light first thing when you wake up, you're telling your body it's the start of the day. This will kickstart your circadian rhythm. First, it will give you energy. Second, you'll find yourself more tired and ready for sleep 14-16 hours later - as nature designed.

4 ways of blasting your eyes with light in the morning:

i) Get an alarm that uses light to wake up. The light gradually gets brighter until it's time to ring the alarm. Helps softly shift the body from its sleep.

ii) Use Re-timer glasses, which are "glasses" that blast your eyes with blue light. Matt's a big fan of these, especially when traveling.

iii) Light earbuds such as Human Charger. These are literally like audio earbuds that you plug into your ears, but instead, they light directly into your brain via your ear canal.

iv) The Sun. Never stare directly into the sun. But waking up, going outside, and looking into the sky is the original way to kickstart your brain in the morning.

One more tip as far as lighting goes, remove all fluorescent lighting from the home and install full-spectrum lighting. It is amazing how this subtle shift can make a big impact on well-being.[180] [181] [182]

Our brains and bodies have evolved on a simple circadian design for millions of years. Light tells the body to wake up. Darkness tells the body to go to sleep. The point is, our bodies aren't designed for the bombardment of blue lights coming from our screens and light bulbs. You're basically recreating nature's pattern by using these technology strategies. We're using biohacking technology to undo the negative consequences of modern technology.

Sleep BiOptimizer #2: Temperature

Temperature

Optimizing the temperature could be the #1 sleep optimizer. Your body WAKES UP when it's too hot. It's another part of the daily circadian rhythm that evolved because of the warmth of the day and the coldness of the night.

If you live in a hot humid climate like Panama, you need to sleep with air conditioners. The question is, is a cold room good enough?

For most people, it's not. Matt used to lose 3-4 lbs of water while he slept despite sleeping in air-conditioned rooms. Why? Because the heat gets trapped between the body, the bedsheets, and the mattress. The body temperature rises and the body begins to sweat. The sheets get damp and the body tosses and turns. It's a massive sleep disrupter.

Fortunately, modern technology has solved this problem. We strongly recommend getting a ChiliPad or Ooler. It's one of the best investments you'll ever make in your sleep. Best of all, if you have a partner, you can get a dual-zone and control each side's temperature.

180 Walls, H. L., Walls, K. L., & Benke, G. (2011). Eye disease resulting from increased use of fluorescent lighting as a climate change mitigation strategy. *American journal of public health, 101*(12), 2222–2225. https://doi.org/10.2105/AJPH.2011.300246
181 L. Morrow, B., & M. Kanakri, S. (2018). The impact of fluorescent and led lighting on students attitudes and behavior in the classroom. *Advances In Pediatric Research.* https://doi.org/10.24105/apr.2018.5.15
182 Swerdlow, A. J., English, J. S., MacKie, R. M., O'Doherty, C. J., Hunter, J. A., Clark, J., & Hole, D. J. (1988). Fluorescent lights, ultraviolet lamps, and risk of cutaneous melanoma. *BMJ (Clinical research ed.), 297*(6649), 647–650. https://doi.org/10.1136/bmj.297.6649.647

Sleep BiOptimizer #3: No Pressure Points

Your body automatically moves when it senses there's blood constriction. For example, if you sleep on your side on a normal mattress, there will be a lot of pressure on your hips and shoulders. This pressure makes your body toss and turn which prevents you from going into a deep sleep.

Pressure Points

For side sleepers, memory foam is a must to spread out the weight evenly. Memory foam mattresses solve this problem by spreading the pressure evenly throughout your body. However one of the issues with some of the foam mattresses is, it traps body heat. This can be solved with the Chili Pad or Ooler.

Another problem with most memory foams is the off-gassing.

For those reasons, we recommend Essentia mattresses. They are made from organic tree sap and you can find the perfect level of softness and density for your body. Matt has a custom-made Pro Core which has been optimized for him and his wife. This is truly the best of the best.

Here are some general rules for selecting the optimal amount of softness:

i) The heavier you are, the more softness you need. You'll sink deeper and even out the weight. Someone who's lighter naturally doesn't need as much weight distribution.

ii) The wider you are (a man with wide shoulders or a woman with wide hips), the more softness you'll need. If someone's body was perfectly straight, the weight would spread evenly. Someone with wide shoulders or wide hips need more softness to give room for that part of the body to sink into.

iii) The shorter you are, the more softness you need. The opposite is true, if you're tall your weight will naturally be distributed over a larger surface.

For back sleepers, this is less of an issue. The weight naturally spreads over a larger surface. Another good brand for back sleepers is Samina.

Sleep BiOptimizer #4: Consistency and Early

Many people say "Every hour you sleep before midnight is worth 2 hours." There's some truth to this. But it's a bit more complex.

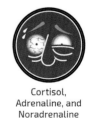

Cortisol, Adrenaline, and Noradrenaline

If you don't go to bed before a certain time (as determined by your circadian rhythm and chronotype), you'll experience a second wind.[183] Back in the days before technology, the only reasons you would stay awake would be either to hunt or protect

---

[183] Weissbluth, M. (1999). *Healthy sleep habits, happy child.* Ballantine Publishing Group.

your tribe. In order to do those things effectively, you need adrenaline and noradrenaline.

If you miss your body's ideal sleep window, the body starts pumping out adrenaline and noradrenaline. This can lead to insomnia.

One thing that will absolutely wreck your sleep is cortisol, adrenaline, and noradrenaline - the body's hormonal and neuro stimulants. This is why going to bed at the right time is critical.

The Health Destroying Sleep Deprivation Cycle

One of the most health-destroying cycles anyone can experience is the sleep deprivation loop. There are various degrees of this.

Our good friend Luke fell into this vicious cycle in his early 20s. He started using various nootropics and stimulants. After a few months, he could only sleep 90 mins a night. All his health markers were crashing. He started BiOptimizing and after a few months, he was able to recover. In chapter 14 "The Healing System".

The next question is, what's early? The answer: it depends on your chronotype. The book "The Power Of When" breaks down 4 chronotypes.

> Lions: wake up early, goes to bed earlier.
> Wolves: stay up later, wake up later.
> Bears: are between lions and wolves -- the majority of the population.
> Dolphins: the insomniacs and light sleepers.

It makes sense from an evolutionary biology perspective. If everyone was a morning person and slept during the night, it would be bad for night invasions. You needed a night crew to protect the tribe.

You can find out which one you are by going www.ThePowerOfWhenQuiz.com

So "early" changes from person to person. For a lion, early could mean 8 pm. For a bear, it's around 10 pm. For a wolf, it's usually before midnight.

Here's the bottom line, you want to go to bed before the "second wind" kicks in. Once the second wind kicks in, your sleep quality that night will suffer.

The hormonal magic zone when you sleep typically happens from 12 am to 3 am. There's a cascade of vital anti-aging hormones including melatonin, prolactin, and growth hormone that your body will NOT release if you aren't sleeping by that time.

Sleep BiOptimizer #5: Meal Timing

Once Matt started tracking sleep, one of the biggest needle movers was meal timing. If Matt ate close to bedtime, his sleep score and deep sleep crashed. If given adequate time to digest, sleep scores were maximized.

The Full Belly

Here's another quote from health researcher Jack Kruse on this topic, *"The prolactin surge does not happen if the patient has sleep apnea or ate some carbs too close to bedtime. If you eat any carbs and protein within 4 hours of sleep you will never see the prolactin surge because any spike in insulin turns off this critical release."*

You shouldn't feel anything lingering in your stomach when you hit the sack. You should feel like you have an empty stomach.

On the flip side, the ideal is not to go to bed hungry. If your ghrelin (the hunger hormone) is growling, it will be hard to fall asleep. What works well is to eat a hearty supper with lots of protein and some fats. That will slow down digestion.

Powermove: Stop Eating 4-6 Hours Before Bedtime

The other Powermove is to use digestive aids like MassZymes, P3OM, and HCL Breakthrough. This will breakdown the food plus maximize your absorption and assimilation of the nutrients.

Sleep BiOptimizer #6: Downshift from the Crazy Beta Brain Train

The brain is always producing various electrical waves depending on what state it's in. Most people are trapped in a beta brain wave state of mind. This is a surefire way to destroy sleep quality. This is the root problem for almost all insomniacs.

Crazy Beta
Brain Train

Mastering Your Brain Waves

There are five major groups of brainwaves. Three of them are on the healing side, and two are more on the fight, flight, or freeze side.

GAMMA WAVES (35 HZ to 100 HZ+): The fastest waves are gamma. When doing EEG analysis on Zen monk masters, gamma is their dominant wave. Gamma is an incredibly high spiritual state. You experience a universal connection with a higher power. However, it can be very taxing on the nervous system. There is a physical cost to it. Not ideal to ramp up gamma before bed.

BETA WAVES (12 HZ TO 30 HZ): With beta, we're engaged, we're focused, we're thinking. If beta goes too high in the wrong parts of the brain, the person experiences anxiety. As discussed earlier, the majority of people are stuck in beta. This is the state many people refer to as "The monkey brain". This is the crazy beta brain train that can create endless streams of thoughts. This is where you can feel your brain is trapped on a hamster wheel. This is one of the greatest destroyers of sleep. It's critical to downshift from this state into...

ALPHA WAVES (8 HZ TO 12 HZ): When you start slowing your brain waves down from beta, you'll enter alpha once you get between 8-12 Hz. Alpha is relaxed and alert. A great first goal for meditators is to reach this state. To maximize sleep, doing a 5 to 20-minute meditation in order to move the brain waves into alpha can do wonders for sleep quality.

THETA WAVES (4 HZ TO 7 HZ): Then if you slow your brain waves down even more to four to seven Hertz, you'll enter theta. This is a much slower and deeper state. This is a fantastic state for visualization. Everyone hits this state at least twice a day. Once when you're falling asleep and once when you wake up. Those states are referred to as hypnagogic (when you fall asleep) or hypnopompic (when you wake up). It's the state where you're slightly aware of your dream.

DELTA WAVES (0.5 HZ TO 4 HZ): And then if you slow it down even more, between zero and four Hz, you'll enter delta. Delta is what we go down to when we hit stage 4 sleep called "deep sleep". Almost all of the healing in your body happens in this sleep phase. Your growth hormone, your testosterone, and most of your rejuvenating, healing hormones get produced in delta sleep. This is also when a lot of your learning happens. This is the foundation of high-quality sleep.

On the fight, flight, or freeze side, we have beta and gamma. On the healing and recovery side, we have alpha, theta, and delta.

Brain Waves and Sleep

The brain remains active during sleep, and each stage of sleep has brain waves that accompany it.

- Stage 1: Alpha waves begin being replaced by theta waves as one transitions from relaxation to sleep. Sleep is light and easily disturbed.

- Stage 2: Brain waves slow down as alpha activity ceases completely and theta waves predominate.

- Stages 3 and 4: Brain activity slows down as delta waves occur. This is the magic zone for rejuvenation and recovery.

- Stage 5 (REM): During the rapid eye movement (REM) stage, the muscles become temporarily paralyzed, and the eyes move quickly. The pattern of brain waves is similar to that in stages 1 and 2, although the sleeper is in a deeper state of sleep.

  According to Dr. Michael J Breus "The Sleep Doctor", *"People with insomnia showed less powerful alpha-wave activity and more powerful beta-wave activity.*

- *With eyes open, people with insomnia displayed less power in alpha waves in at least two different areas of the brain, within the frontal and temporal lobes.*

- *With eyes closed, people with insomnia showed more powerful beta waves globally throughout the brain. "*

So if you can boost your alpha brain waves and lower your beta brain waves before sleep, you will improve your sleep quality dramatically. Serotonin levels in the brain also maintain the ratio between slow brain waves (so-called delta–theta activity) and alpha brain waves.

Serotonin is critical for melatonin. The precursor to melatonin is serotonin, a neurotransmitter that itself is derived from the amino acid tryptophan. Within the pineal gland, serotonin is acetylated and then methylated to yield melatonin. It is Matt's theory that by getting into an alpha state, you'll boost your serotonin and improve your sleep quality. Magnesium Breakthrough can do wonders in this department. Take 2-3 caps, an hour Before bed will kick start the serotonin-melatonin cycle.

We will cover brain waves in greater depth in chapter 15 the "BiOptimizing Your Brain" and discuss ways of optimizing them.

Powermove: Shift Your Brain Before Bed

It's wise to downshift your brain before bed. Here are some ways you can do this:

1 - Meditate for 5-20 minutes before bed.

2 - Another great Powermove is to do a "Gratitude List". Gratitude is one of the most effective ways to boost alpha brain waves. Do a gratitude list and spend a few minutes feeling that gratitude in your heart. Just close your eyes and feel each thing you're grateful for in your heart.

3 - Brain Dumps: if you're the type of person with racing thoughts and non-stop creative ideas, spending time every night dumping your thoughts on paper can do wonders for quieting the mind. Just grab a paper and pen and keep writing until your brain runs dry.

The next chapter will cover another critical piece to getting good sleep by optimizing your nervous system. This will make it far easier to downshift your brain at night because if you're trapped in a fight-flight-freeze state, it will destroy your sleep. We will cover this in chapter 14.

Sleep Supplements

Let's divide these supplements into 2 categories:

1 - Uppers: stimulates the nervous system.
2 - Relaxers: downregulates the nervous system.

Obviously, you want to minimize and eliminate the uppers 6 to 12 hours before bedtime. The exact timing depends on how fast your body metabolizes these compounds. For example, take caffeine. If you're a slow caffeine metabolizer, one cup afternoon can disrupt sleep significantly. If you're a fast caffeine metabolizer, you can drink an espresso and pass out.

Uppers include:

1 - Caffeine, including coffee, teas, energy drinks, and pre-workouts.
2 - Nicotine.
3 - Adderall, Ritalin, and Vyvanse.
4 - THC (sativa).

A lot of people are pushing their adrenal glands to the limit and beyond by overdosing on caffeine and other stimulants.[184] Vaping and other nicotine sources are at record highs.

We're not here to knock these or tell anyone they shouldn't consume these. Our message is to manage your nervous system. Balance the yin and yang.

The other strategy is to ramp down the nervous system by using relaxers in the evening and weekends.

Relaxers:

1 - Magnesium
2 - L-Theanine
3 - Lavender Oil
4 - Ashwagandha
5 - Reishi
6 - CBD

All of these should be tried to see how your body responds.

---

[184] *Energy Drinks Market Size, Share & Demand | Industry Analysis 2026.* Allied Market Research. (2019). Retrieved 2 October 2020, from https://www.alliedmarketresearch.com/energy-drink-market.

Powermove: Use L-Theanine to Optimize Your Nervous System

Another extremely effective sleep enhancer is taking 100-400 mg of L-Theanine before bed. L-Theanine can also be stacked with your coffee for great results. It will extend the caffeine's effects and smooth out the adrenal response. L-Theanine boosts alpha brain waves and as we explained earlier it can improve sleep quality big time.

Conclusion

High quality sleep is perhaps the most powerful biological optimizer. It improves everything from aesthetics by growing lean muscle mass and burning body fat. Sleep enhances your performance by getting your body and mind in its best state. And upgrades your health on countless levels.

Chapter 12

Biological Optimizer #3: The Power of Getting Lean and Muscular

In this chapter, you will learn:

- **The #1 problem with most approaches to "losing weight".**

- Why it's not about pounds and what to focus on instead.

- **How to increase your metabolic rate and transform your body faster.**

- And much more...

Lean Muscle Mass

Lower levels of body fat and optimal levels of lean muscle mass are two of the main determinants of healthspan and lifespan. They expand all 3 sides of the BiOptimization Triangle.

It improves how you look. It improves your health and it improves your mental and physical performance.

We're not going to spend a lot of time discussing the aesthetics of lean muscle mass. That is a highly personal matter. It ranges from guys wanting to look like bodybuilders to guys just wanting to look lean and fit. Some women want to hop on stage with bikinis and some women just want to look and feel good in their clothes.

The purpose of this chapter is to drive home the health and performance benefits of lean muscle mass and lower body fat. It's to help you understand how it will improve the quality of your life especially as you get older.

What Should Your Goal Be?

Here are the various health ranges for body fat and FFMI (FFMI stands for Fat-Free Mass Index). To calculate it, take your fat-free lean body mass and divide by your height in inches.

Ideal Ranges for Men

Men Range	Body Fat Levels	FFMI (Fat-Free Mass Index)
Unhealthy Danger Zone	35%+	Below 14
Unhealthy	25-34%	15-17
Average/Healthy	18-25%	18-19
Optimal/Athletic	8-18%	20-27
Maximization Zone (Danger)	7% or less	Over 28

Some key points on this chart:

- Past 27 FFMI, you're entering the Maximization Zone and it will almost certainly require steroids, testosterone, and other enhancers.[185]

- Body fat percentage-wise, less is better up to a point. Below 8%, the body will go into fight-flight-freeze mode unless you're a genetic freak.

- Every person has an optimal body fat range depending on their genetics and life history. The body has a set point. When you try to push the body past that point, expect the body to start fighting back. This can create severe metabolic damage and other health problems. For some men, that will be 18% and others it will be 9%.

Ideal Ranges for Women

Women Range	Body Fat Levels	FFMI (Fat-Free Mass Index)
Unhealthy Danger Zone	40%+	Below 11
Unhealthy	30-39%	12-14
Average/Healthy	23-29%	15-17
Optimal/Athletic	11-22%	18-22
Maximization Zone (Danger)	10% or less	Over 23

Some key points on this chart:

- This chart was created by examining the stats of fitness competitors as well as female pro bodybuilders.

- Past 23 FFMI, you're entering the Maximization Zone and it will almost certainly require steroids, testosterone, and other enhancers.

- Just like men, women have an optimal body fat range depending on their genetics and life history. For some women, that will be 11% and others it will be 22%.

Body fat percentage-wise, less is better up to a point. Women need a higher percentage of body fat than men. For most women, body fat levels below 10% can lead to health problems unless they're genetic freaks. For women, this can lead to a host of serious health issues including hormonal problems and metabolic damage.

---

[185] Kouri, E. M., Pope, H. G., Jr, Katz, D. L., & Oliva, P. (1995). Fat-free mass index in users and nonusers of anabolic-androgenic steroids. *Clinical journal of sport medicine : official journal of the Canadian Academy of Sport Medicine, 5*(4), 223–228. https://doi.org/10.1097/00042752-199510000-00003

How to Lose Excess Body Fat

Losing excess body fat is very simple: burn more calories than you're consuming. This is what the majority of fat loss experts will tell you. Is that helpful? Not really.

Is it easy to lose body fat? No, it's one of the hardest things anyone can do, especially when you consider long term fat loss success. Only 3% of people succeed in losing excess body fat and keeping it off. That's right, 97% of people haven't been able to do it successfully.

The reasons why and the solutions to these reasons are far too complex to fully address in this book. However, we want to cover the fundamentals to give you a starting point and give you some direction.

The Core Reason Why People Fail With Weight Loss Long Term

The body has one main goal: SURVIVAL. The human body evolved over billions of years to maximize its chances of survival.

If we took a time machine back to caveman days, there wasn't an abundance of convenience stores and fast food restaurants. Food had to be hunted or gathered. There were no fruits and vegetables during the long, hard winter months. Humans could go days or weeks without any food.

In order to maximize the odds of survival, the body created many self-defense mechanisms. And these self-defense mechanisms are why people fail with their weight loss objectives long term.

Imagine a 150 lbs caveman, named Carl, with a body fat percentage of 10%. This means he has about 7% body fat percentage (which is around 24,500 calories) he can lose before his body starts shutting down. The male body will start shutting down around 3%. This means he has around 24,500 "survival calories" left.

Assuming Carl is burning 2,500 calories a day as he's trying to gather or hunt food, he has about 10 days left for survival, which is NOT very long in the long winter months.

However, there's a twist to this story: the body evolved to protect us from this situation. The body will lower metabolism in order to create a better probability of survival. If the body was only burning 1,250 calories a day, it would double the amount of time Carl The Caveman could survive.

Here's a short list of the survival mechanisms the body uses in extended calorie deprivation:

1 - Lowers testosterone
2 - Lowers leptin
3 - Lowers thyroid function
4 - Increases ghrelin (which increases hunger)
5 - Lowers N.E.A.T., which is useless motion (non-exercise activity thermogenesis)
6 - Burn lean muscle mass

The problem is, we still have the same programming that Carl The Caveman has today.

When Matt was getting ready for his marriage, he wanted to lose an additional 15 lbs to look his best. Matt had already lost over 30 lbs in the 2 years prior. Matt PUSHED HARD. He was doing sprints up hills in the jungle and cut his calories further.

Matt did lose the 15 lbs, but then THE HUNGER came. Matt felt hungry for 2 years after that and regained most of the lost weight. It was a huge learning lesson. The body increased ghrelin in order to maximize the odds of survival.

So what's the core principle for weight loss?

IT'S: MAKE THE BODY FEEL SAFE.

This is why refeeds, diet breaks and reverse dieting are 3 critical tools for people wanting to lose body fat permanently, safely, and not go through the yo-yo dieting insanity.

Reasons Why Most Fat Loss Fails:

1 - Dieting too fast.

"12-week transformations" and other short-term diet goals are one of the main culprits for these weight-loss failures. Going back to Carl the Caveman's example, if you're losing too much body fat, too fast, it will activate its survival mechanisms and that's when you're basically screwed.

Can you lose body fat quickly? Yes, however, diet breaks should be incorporated every 2-4 weeks to let the body know that IT'S SAFE.

Do NOT sacrifice the future for today. As an example, if you've got 50 lbs to lose, give yourself a year, even two. It will make the journey more enjoyable and maximize the odds of success.

2 - No diet breaks and refeeds.

Diet breaks, which means eating at maintenance for a week or two, can make all the difference in the world for extended fat loss journeys.

Another option is to eat two days of higher calories a week. As long as your weekly calories are in a deficit, you'll be losing body fat. Make sure to track your overall calories and not overeat on the weekends. You can easily blow five days of progress in two days.

3 - Following an unsustainable diet.

In order to be successful FOR LIFE, you must find a nutritional philosophy that you can follow. Anyone with a bit of willpower can cut calories using drastic measures, but the real question is: *"what's next?"* What are you going to do AFTER?

The real challenge isn't the weight loss, it's the life-long maintenance.

4 - Not following an exercise program that they enjoy.

Exercise, both movement and resistance training, are critical components to a successful weight-loss and weight-maintenance program. The only way you're going to stick with it is finding something that you enjoy doing and make it a habit.

5 - Not resolving underlying emotional issues.

Most people who are overweight use food as a drug. Food has drug-like effects both on dopamine and serotonin. People with food issues use food to escape the emotional pain or boredom they're feeling.

The answer to this is to do a deep inventory of emotional issues and systematically clear them using tools such as EFT, forgiveness work, neurofeedback, EMDR, or other modalities.

6 - Not tracking things: food calories and macros, sleep, exercise.

You can't improve what you don't measure. It's critical to create feedback loops (more on this in the chapter on Biological Optimization Process).

It's easy to lose weight in the beginning by making a few simple diet or exercise changes. However, this won't last forever. As you go further down the path, precise changes and decisions need to be made. It becomes a guessing game if you don't track.

7 - No coaching or accountability in place.

Coaching and accountability are critical for success. We go in great depth in the "Jedi Council" appendix. A great coach will help motivate you, solve your problems and create a great strategy.

8 - Low-quality sleep.

Low-quality sleep makes losing weight multiple times harder. Your hunger hormones go up, your cravings increase, you start burning lean muscle mass instead of body fat, your will power goes down, and your fat-burning hormones (HGH and testosterone) go down.

Make sure to implement the tips and strategies from the sleep chapter.

9 - Not addressing other health problems.

Other underlying health problems such as hormonal issues, gut issues, fatty liver and much more can make losing body fat a much tougher journey. Work with your Jedi Health Council to address these issues.

10 - Losing mental vigilance.

It's important to always be vigilant. It's easy to lose awareness and start slowly regaining the lost weight. It's easy to stop tracking calories and macros and start increasing calories. It's easy to drop exercise habits and default to old habits. Once you lose mental vigilance, it's usually the beginning of the end.

The answer is: don't drop your guard. Weigh yourself EVERY DAY. Get a body fat scan once or twice a year. Join health communities. Get blood work twice a year. Hire coaches. Get accountability buddies. Find fun workout partners. Stack the odds of success in your favor.

By following and incorporating the Powermoves and advice in this book, you should be able to lower your body fat over time. If you're serious about losing a lot of body fat, we suggest joining our coaching program at www.bioptimizers.com/coaching.

Lean Muscle Mass and Lifespan

First, let's discuss the lifespan benefits of muscle mass.

Professor Claudio Gil Araújo followed 3,878 people for 6.5 years. The participants in the weakest quartile had a risk of dying that was 10 to 13 times higher than that of those in the top 3rd or 4th quartile. As you get older, the quality of your life becomes highly correlated by your lean muscle mass and strength.[186]

---

[186] de Brito, L., Ricardo, D., de Araújo, D., Ramos, P., Myers, J., & de Araújo, C. (2012). Ability to sit and rise from the floor as a predictor of all-cause mortality. *European Journal Of Preventive Cardiology, 21*(7), 892-898. https://doi.org/10.1177/2047487312471759

- Leg strength is what determines if you fall down easily.

- It's what determines if you can cross the street quickly.

- Can you carry your groceries?

- Can you go up and down stairs easily?

Matt saw this firsthand with his own grandfather who lived in his home growing up. He got hit by a car. A couple of years later, he fell down and broke his hip. This was the beginning of the end. Once his mobility went downhill, so did his health. The last few years of his life were spent in agonizing pain. He was literally praying for death. It was a very sad and traumatizing experience to witness.

Now let's discuss its impact on healthspan.

Muscle is alive. It's metabolically active. It burns energy. This keeps your metabolism healthy.

It helps store glucose. This helps prevent blood sugar-related health problems. Here's what Dr. Gabrielle Lyons, who calls muscle "the organ of longevity" has to say about this:[187] [188]

"Muscle plays a central role in whole-body protein metabolism by serving as the principal reservoir for amino acids to maintain protein synthesis in vital tissues and organs in the absence of amino acid absorption from the gut and by providing hepatic gluconeogenic precursors. Furthermore, altered muscle metabolism plays a key role in the genesis, and therefore the prevention, of many common pathologic conditions and chronic diseases."

Your organs need amino acids for repair. It can go get them from your muscle mass. There are massive blood sugar management benefits of lean muscle mass.

We could write an entire book on the health benefits of lean muscle mass. Hopefully, this was enough to "sell you" on it.

Here's some great news: it doesn't matter how old you are, if you're a man or woman, you can build muscle mass. Tons of research has been done with elderly people and they can build muscle and gain strength.

[187] Lyon, G. (2018). High-quality protein is essential for healthier muscles. Retrieved 2 October 2020, from https://www.arla-foodsingredients.com/the-whey-and-protein-blog/health/high-quality-protein-is-essential-for-healthier-muscles/.
[188] Wolfe R. R. (2006). The underappreciated role of muscle in health and disease. *The American journal of clinical nutrition, 84*(3), 475–482. https://doi.org/10.1093/ajcn/84.3.475

Powermove: Start Resistance Training and Never Stop

Our advice is to start now and make it a non-negotiable health habit. Here's more good news: the minimum effective dose is 3 times a week in as little as 20 to 30 minutes per session.

That means you can experience the majority of the benefits laid out in this chapter in 60 to 90 minutes a week. It's one of the highest returns on investments you'll ever do health-wise.

The key is, it must be challenging resistance. One challenging set of weight-bearing squats has infinitely more benefits than doing 10 sets on Suzanne Somers' Thighmaster.

The solution is simple: resistance training combined with proper nutrification (which will cover later) will add decades to your healthspan and most likely improve your lifespan.

Chapter 13

Biological Optimizer #4: Life Is Movement

In this chapter, you will learn:

- **Going beyond exercise: movement that transforms your body and cellular health.**

- How to workout in a way that removes toxins and reverses aging.

- **Our favorite exercises for fat loss (without stressing out your nervous system).**

- And much more...

Movement

Aristotle once said, "*Life requires movement.*" He nailed it. Movement has incredible benefits on all 3 sides of the BiOptimization Triangle. We've separated "Movement" from "Build Lean Muscle Mass" because it is different and it does warrant its own focus.

As far as improving lifespan and healthspan, movement is one of the most powerful game-changers. As far as anti-aging effects, here's a quote from a research paper from Rebelo-Marques and co. called "Aging Hallmarks: The Benefits of Physical Exercise".[189]

"Exercise should be seen as a polypill, which improves the health-related quality of life and functional capabilities while mitigating physiological changes and comorbidities associated with aging."

So yes movement does positively affect all 9 of the drivers of aging.

Health: Movement and Lifespan

Association of Daily Step Count and Step Intensity With Mortality Among US Adults, backed up this theory published by JAMA (Journal Of American Medical Association) revealing the data.[190]

---

189 Rebelo-Marques, A., De Sousa Lages, A., Andrade, R., Ribeiro, C. F., Mota-Pinto, A., Carrilho, F., & Espregueira-Mendes, J. (2018). Aging Hallmarks: The Benefits of Physical Exercise. *Frontiers in endocrinology, 9,* 258. https://doi.org/10.3389/fendo.2018.00258

190 Saint-Maurice, P. F., Troiano, R. P., Bassett, D. R., Jr, Graubard, B. I., Carlson, S. A., Shiroma, E. J., Fulton, J. E., & Matthews, C. E. (2020). Association of Daily Step Count and Step Intensity With Mortality Among US Adults. JAMA, 323(12), 1151–1160. https://doi.org/10.1001/jama.2020.1382

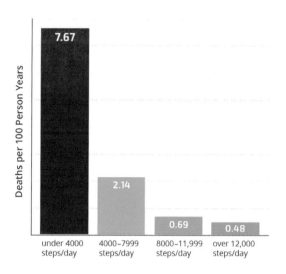

Health: Movement and Vitality

"Sitting is the new smoking" is something you may have heard in the last few years. This is a bit inaccurate. "Not moving is the new smoking" is more accurate.

There's nothing extra dangerous about "sitting". However, after 30 minutes of inactivity, a cascade of negative biological reactions begin to occur. So it doesn't matter if you're lying, standing, squatting, or sitting, lack of movement is the problem.

Shifting from the 5 Postures

Fortunately, the answer is simple: change positions and move every half hour. Cycle through all 5 positions: sitting, standing, lying down, squatting, and walking.

Go from sitting to standing. Take a walk to the bathroom. Go get a glass of water. Squat down for three minutes. Go play with your pets. MOVE. According to the research, you only need to move one minute every half hour.

Squatting all the way down is very powerful. It helps stretch out your legs and lower back. It helps you find tight spots in your body that you can work on later.

Find Your Movement Passion and Make it a Habit

The first key is to find a movement that you LOVE to do. We want to connect with the child within us. Children aren't counting steps and "trying to do exercise". They play. They have fun. Let's keep that playful passion alive. It doesn't matter if you love to surf, do yoga, play sports, do martial arts, or run. MOVE.

The more important key is to make it a habit. If you're going to choose surfing, schedule it 3 times a week. If you're going to play sports, make sure you're playing all year round. We've seen the pattern hundreds of times with our clients. As they get older and "life gets in the way", these passions fall by the wayside. The sedentary "Netflix and chill" lifestyle takes over.

Brain and Movement

The effects movement has on the brain are epic. In Mason Currey's book "Daily Rituals: How Artists Work" he breaks down the 24-hour cycles and habits of the greatest minds of all time. Virtually all of them have a walking and thinking habit. Walking helps synchronize the right and left brain which can be potent for problem-solving.

Steve Jobs, the late co-founder of Apple, was known for his walking meetings. Facebook's Mark Zuckerberg has also been seen holding meetings on foot. Bill Gates loves to walk and talk.

Here are more brain benefits of walking and movement: [191]

Research has shown that just 20 mins of exercise or walking can cut the risk of developing depression by a third. Research has also shown that walking in nature has far more benefits than walking on a treadmill in a gym.

Powermove: The 3-Day Nature Reset

Every month go on a 3-day nature reboot. Take a long weekend and go to a hotel on the beach. Go enjoy a cabin in the woods. It does wonders for your mind, performance, and health.

Why? David Strayer has the answer.[192]

[191] Schuch, F. B., Vancampfort, D., Firth, J., Rosenbaum, S., Ward, P. B., Silva, E. S., Hallgren, M., Ponce De Leon, A., Dunn, A. L., Deslandes, A. C., Fleck, M. P., Carvalho, A. F., & Stubbs, B. (2018). Physical Activity and Incident Depression: A Meta-Analysis of Prospective Cohort Studies. *The American journal of psychiatry, 175*(7), 631–648. https://doi.org/10.1176/appi.ajp.2018.17111194

[192] Publishing, H. (2016). *Need a quick brain boost? Take a walk - Harvard Health.* Harvard Health. Retrieved 2 October 2020, from https://www.health.harvard.edu/mind-and-mood/need-a-quick-brain-boost-take-a-walk.

David Strayer brings people into nature and wires their brain to EEG machines and shows them the profound changes that happen in just 3 days. Here's an excerpt from a National Geographic article.

"Our brains, he says, aren't tireless three-pound machines; they're easily fatigued. When we slow down, stop the busywork, and take in beautiful natural surroundings, not only do we feel restored, but our mental performance improves too. Strayer has demonstrated as much with a group of Outward Bound participants, who performed 50 percent better on creative problem-solving tasks after three days of wilderness backpacking. The three-day effect, he says, is a kind of cleaning of the mental windshield that occurs when we've been immersed in nature long enough."

Overall improvements in cognition and reaction time have been measured and proven in several experiments. All it takes is 20 to 30 minutes of movement.[193]

A survey in the UK found that all it took to reach a natural high is nine minutes and 44 seconds. One of our favorite sayings comes from the legendary bodybuilder, Tom Platz *"Any problems you have in life, the iron always saves you."* From a neurochemical level that is accurate. If you feel stressed and frustrated, and then have a good workout, you'll have a totally brand new perspective afterwards.

Remember this: there are no bad workouts. Only good ones and great ones.[194]

BDNF (brain-derived neurotrophic factors) is the brain's natural fertilizer. BDNF helps your brain grow new neurons and cells. All it takes is one 30 min walk to boost your BDNF. We will talk in greater depth later about all the powerful benefits of BDNF in chapter 14.[195]

You can lower your fatigue by 65% by integrating movement into your life. Remember, when your body doesn't move there's a cascade of problems that occur. Blood flow slows down. Oxygen levels drop. Mitochondria (your cell's energy factories) die and become weak. This is critical for mental focus and drive.[196]

Research has shown that adults who walked 40 minutes, three times a week had brain growth in their hippocampus. This improves your spatial memory. Hippocampus is also one of the areas of the brain that produces new neurons from stem cells. It's noteworthy that the hippocampal function declines with age. Walking can be a simple antidote to this.[197]

---

[193] *Runners' high kicks in sooner than you think.* Wiggle Blog. (2018). Retrieved 2 October 2020, from https://blog.wiggle.co.uk/runners%E2%80%99-high-kicks-sooner-you-think.

[194] Morais, V., Tourino, M., Almeida, A., Albuquerque, T., Linhares, R. C., Christo, P. P., Martinelli, P. M., & Scalzo, P. L. (2018). A single session of moderate intensity walking increases brain-derived neurotrophic factor (BDNF) in the chronic post-stroke patients. *Topics in stroke rehabilitation, 25*(1), 1–5. https://doi.org/10.1080/10749357.2017.1373500

[195] *Low-intensity exercise reduces fatigue symptoms by 65 percent, study finds* - UGA Today. UGA Today. (2008). Retrieved 2 October 2020, from https://news.uga.edu/low-intensity-exercise-reduces-fatigue-symptoms-by-65-percent-study-finds/.

[196] Colcombe, S., & Kramer, A. F. (2003). Fitness effects on the cognitive function of older adults: a meta-analytic study. Psychological science, 14(2), 125–130. https://doi.org/10.1111/1467-9280.t01-1-01430

[197] Oppezzo, M., & Schwartz, D. L. (2014). Give your ideas some legs: the positive effect of walking on creative thinking. Journal of experimental psychology. *Learning, memory, and cognition, 40*(4), 1142–1152. https://doi.org/10.1037/a0036577

Want a 60% boost in creativity? If you answered "YES", then walk. In several experiments involving 176 students and adults, creativity was measured and the results were impressive. Those that walked (from 5 to 16 minutes) had 60% more creativity on divergent thinking tests and complex analogy tests.[198]

CBS News reported in 2017 that a recent study discovered twenty minutes of walking increased cerebral blood flow. And, like with any major organ, increasing circulation is super important to the health of both your brain and body. As the website Brain MD Health explained, blood flow helps to bring "nutrients to your cells, and takes away toxins."

Lymphatic Benefits

Movement also activates the lymphatic vessels. Unlike blood circulation which is triggered by the heart, the lymphatic system does not have an organ to pump it into action and must rely completely on your movement and muscle contractions to help it perform its function.

A healthy lymphatic system wards off infections and even prevents cancer. That's because it is responsible for scavenging for excess water and protein leaked from capillaries, abnormal cells, particles, viruses, and bacteria which then becomes lymph fluid and passes through lymph nodes to kill any potentially harmful matter.[199]

The main lymph vessels run up the legs, arms, and torso so a power walk can be a great way to improve your lymph health and boost immunity.

The Top 5 Ways to Move

Here are our top 5 suggestions for movement:

1 - Walking

Walking is the king of movement. It's free, it's accessible anywhere on Earth and it produces great benefits. Walking in or around nature is ideal. Walking is a great low-stress fat-burner (you can burn up to 600 calories doing 10,000 steps) and does wonders for the synchronization of the brain.

---

[198] *Low-intensity exercise reduces fatigue symptoms by 65 percent, study finds* - UGA Today. UGA Today. (2008). Retrieved 2 October 2020, from https://news.uga.edu/low-intensity-exercise-reduces-fatigue-symptoms-by-65-percent-study-finds/.
[199] Moore, J. E., Jr, & Bertram, C. D. (2018). Lymphatic System Flows. *Annual review of fluid mechanics, 50*, 459–482. https://doi.org/10.1146/annurev-fluid-122316-045259

---

2 - Rebounding

Rebounding is unique to other movements because of its powerful lymphatic benefits. Put on some great tunes and start bouncing and dancing for a fun, powerful workout.

3 - Swimming

Swimming is powerful for 2 reasons. First, it lowers gravity which is great for people with bad joints. Second, it produces heat loss which is another way to burn calories.

4 - Yoga

Yoga is powerful and unique due to its parasympathetic activation and its stretching benefits.

5 - Your Favorite Sports

Whatever your favorite sport is, should be your main movement. It's hard to beat the power of passion when it comes to motivation and inspiration.

Conclusion

Movement is critical for your body and your brain. All it takes is 10 to 30 min walks. Remember the most important thing is to make this an unconscious habit. Not to mention the powerful blood sugar "10-minute walk" technique after meals.

Chapter 14

Biological Optimizer #5: BiOptimizing Your Nervous System

In this chapter, you will learn:

- **How to make your body twice as resilient to stress and trauma.**

- The #1 overlooked factor in your mental health and how to feel good more often.

- **Balancing the demands of high performance with your body's need to relax.**

- And much more...

Optimizing Your
Nervous System

Perhaps the most visceral system that directly affects us on a daily basis is the nervous system. Yet it is one of the most ignored systems in the body. The good news is, it's one of the systems you have the most influence and control over. That's what this chapter is about. In terms of the quality of your life, understanding how to optimize your nervous system is one of the most important factors.

The High Performer's Dilemma: Pushing the Lines

Part of being a high performer is to find that balance between high performance and not burning out. For those of us that have purposes and missions that were committed to, we want our cake and we want to eat it too. We want to be a superhuman because we have to manifest our visions. The risk is that the quality of our health and lives can go downhill if we don't learn to manage our nervous system.

Wade experienced a very deep level of burnout a couple of years ago. Here's the story in his own words:

"I was in Bali, which was almost a dozen hours difference time zone wise from most of my team. I decided to start a new company. I've got BiOptimizers which is a rapidly growing company.

I'm doing mornings with one business partner, very early in the day. And I'm staying up till like 3:00 am or 4:00 am. I'd sleep three hours, wake up, do one business, go for a massage in the afternoon, come back, go to work again, sleep for an hour and a half, wake up and then work the evenings.

After a couple of months of that, I really started paying the price. Energy and mental performance were dropping. To compensate, I increased my caffeine intake. I used my nootropics to help my brain focus.

I "felt" like my brain was laser because I felt the adrenaline from the caffeine and nootropics. However, this energy was coming from pushing my adrenal glands to the max. This wasn't sustainable. It's like paying your mortgage off with your credit card. I was robbing Peter to pay Paul.

Then the unexpected happened. There were a bunch of crises that came up. I had a problem in my growth business and that was a serious challenge with my partner, and that's the event that took me out.

That's when I ran out of gas and I was totally physiologically burned out. It didn't matter how much caffeine I was taking, it wasn't helping. My adrenal glands weren't functioning. I was in an unresourceful psychological state and dark, negative emotional place. I told Matt 'I'm in a living hell'."

Fortunately, Wade was able to recover using the principles and techniques in this chapter.
Read this chapter carefully and more importantly implement the strategies and tactics in this chapter if you want to avoid this. What we're really talking about is managing your nervous system for maximum success, health, and happiness.

Cycles of Intensity and Recovery

The key lesson of this chapter is to cycle between intensity and recovery. Those that master this, can become high performers and maintain that for most if not all of their lives. Those that don't will have a spurt of high performance, followed by a steep decline in performance ending with a brutal burnout. Some burnouts take years to recover from. Some people become traumatized psychologically by the pain of the burnout and recoil from intensity for the rest of their lives.

A 2 Gear System: Fight-Flight-Freeze or Heal

Your nervous system is made of two systems:

1 - Parasympathetic: also known as the "healing system".
2 - Sympathetic: also known as "fight, flight or freeze" a.k.a. "The survival system".

The Survival System

The sympathetic nervous system evolved to save us from dangerous or stressful situations. A flood of survival hormones cranks the body's alertness and heart rate, sending extra blood to the muscles. Breathing speeds up to deliver more oxygen to the brain, and an infusion of glucose is shot into the bloodstream for a quick energy boost.

This system is designed to mobilize us or help us defend ourselves against threats: deadly animals, other humans, etc...

Let's just go back to the caveman days. There's a saber tooth tiger chasing you. You need to activate your sympathetic system and hopefully fight or flight kicks in, because if you freeze you're usually dead. To survive you need to run really fast or successfully fight this threat off. If it wasn't for this system, there would be no humans. This system has helped humans survive and thrive over millions of years.

It's intrinsic to being an animal. You can see that in nature. Watch African nature shows. You see this when lion's attack the hyenas and cape buffalos. You'll even see it in bacteria. The bacterium will recoil against a toxic substance. It's fleeing away from it.

One of the key things for us to understand is that anything you believe or feel is a threat will activate this system. This means, if you lose your job and you have economic insecurity, you will feel fear and activate the survival system. Maybe you just launched a marketing campaign that failed, and you feel concerned. Maybe your romantic partner just insulted you and you're scared of being alone.

The average person is caught in a sympathetic loop. When they wake up, they activate their beta brain waves. They check their phones... have a cup of coffee and have food on the run. Then they have a stressful commute to work. They have a long hard day's work and then they do another stressful commute back home. When they get home they spend more time hijacked on their phones and then fall asleep.

The Stressed Out Lifestyle

LOW-QUALITY SLEEP

STIMULANTS

LIFE STRESS

WORKOUTS

WORK

The only time they're parasympathetic is when they fall asleep, and for most of them, it's low quality sleep. They repeat that pattern and they're kind of stuck into this vicious cycle. This person is essentially stuck in fight, flight, or freeze.

The Healing System [200]

The parasympathetic system is what puts your body in a healing state for it to recover, rest, and rejuvenate.

Before the advance in the industrial ages and technologies, we spent far more time in parasympathetic mode. When the sun went down, we went to bed. Our brain's dopamine system wasn't hijacked by apps, porn, games, movies, and shows. There was far less stimulation than there is today. Our brains weren't being fooled by blue light coming from all of these devices.

The danger is when your body becomes dominated by one of these systems. The most common problem is people become trapped in a fight-flight-or-freeze lifestyle. Entrepreneurs and motivated career-driven people easily fall into this trap.

They travel the world, manage multiple products, start new businesses, lead dozens or even hundreds of thousands of people. They constantly learn new skills and systems. Sleep is cut down to make more time for work. Diet is compromised by restaurant meals and other low quality food options. Complex problems arise constantly. High-stress situations and problems come daily.

The Solution

The answer is to consciously shift your mind and body into parasympathetic mode systemically. This means incorporating certain habits and rituals that move you into healing mode.

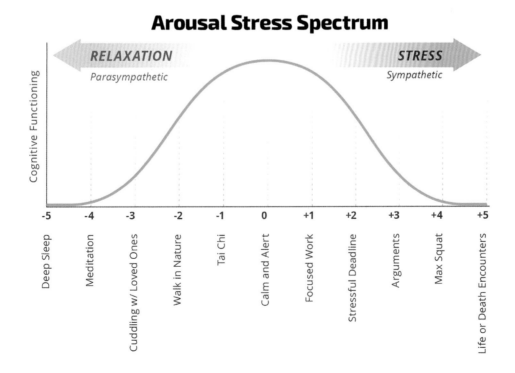

200 *Noyes' Knee Disorders: Surgery, Rehabilitation, Clinical Outcomes.* (2017). https://doi.org/10.1016/c2013-0-18673-4

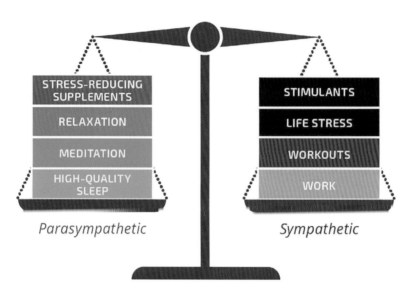

Managing Your Nervous System

Exercise

Let's start with exercise. Exercise is primarily fight or flight. When you're lifting weights or doing CrossFit -- that's a fight or flight response. When you're playing sports, it's a fight or flight response. Even things like running, it's literally flight.

Now on the healing side, there are some exercises that work. One is Tai-Chi and other similar slow type movements that focus on slow breathing. The slow movement and conscious breathing activate the parasympathetic, healing part of your nervous system.

Another great one is yoga. The slower style of yoga is really interesting because it's physically challenging. However, because you're really slowing down the breath it calms down your nervous system.

Meditation

Perhaps the most powerful nervous system shifter is meditation. In minutes, you can shift your state from fight-flight-freeze to calm and relaxed. We will cover various meditation strategies in the next chapter.

Heart Rate Variability

Heart rate variability (HRV) is the most useful data point to manage your nervous system. HRV is the best indicator to see where your nervous system is at. HRV measures the variance between heartbeats. When you inhale, you will typically see a shortening of the time. When you exhale, you'll see a lengthening.

The more stressed you are, the lower your HRV is. The more relaxed you are, the higher your HRV is.

Tools to Measure HRV

For overall NS measurements, we prefer Oura-Ring. It gives you a "Readiness Score" that measures how fried or fresh the nervous system is in the morning. However, for real-time measurements, we prefer Bio-Strap. You can do real-time experiments and measure your HRV. Push a button and two minutes later you get a score.

BiOptimizing Your Neurotransmitters

Here's the fundamental problem from a neurotransmitter perspective: people are taxing their adrenal glands and functioning on adrenaline and noradrenaline.[201] People are tired and wired.

The other big problem from a neurotransmitter perspective is not enough of the good stuff. This section will break down the key neurotransmitters to focus on and simple things you can do to manage them.

Next, let's segway into neurotransmitters.

On the healing side, we have four neurotransmitters:

1 - Serotonin, which makes you feel more relaxed. It gets released when you eat sugar. That's one of the reasons people who suffer from emotional eating, consume a lot of sugar. It makes them feel a little more relaxed.

2 - Endorphins: our body's natural pain killer. It's the rewards you get after a hard workout, running, or eating very hot peppers.

3 - Oxytocin: the love molecule. In the first 12 months when you start dating someone new, there's elevated levels of oxytocin. The biggest boost of oxytocin is when a woman gives birth to a baby through the birth canal. After sex, there's a big oxytocin release. This is why women love cuddling.

4 - Anandamide: the bliss molecule. Anandamide is a type of endocannabinoid — the body's own version of cannabis. Scientists believe that people's enhanced levels of happiness are a direct result of having more anandamide in their system. Ways to boost this include: CBD, exercise, and eating the darkest chocolate possible (major boost if it's raw).

---

[201] TNicola Twilley, G. (2016). *Caffeine: The World's Most Popular Drug.* The Atlantic. Retrieved 2 October 2020, from https://www.theatlantic.com/science/archive/2016/03/worlds-most-popular-drug/474831/.

And then on the sympathetic side:

1 - Adrenaline: Adrenaline (also known as epinephrine) and noradrenaline are two separate but related hormones and neurotransmitters. They are produced in the centre of the adrenal glands. They are released into the bloodstream and serve as chemical mediators, and also convey the nerve impulses to various organs. Key actions of adrenaline include increasing the heart rate, increasing blood pressure, expanding the air passages of the lungs, enlarging the pupils, shifting blood to the muscles, and altering the body's metabolism to maximize blood glucose levels.

2 - A closely related hormone to adrenaline, noradrenaline (also known as norepinephrine), is released primarily from the nerve endings of the sympathetic nervous system. Helps to increase the force of skeletal muscle contractions and the rate and force of contraction of the heart (which increases blood pressure). There is a continuous low level of activity of the sympathetic nervous system resulting in the release of noradrenaline into the circulation, but adrenaline release is only increased at times of acute or intense stress.

3 - Dopamine: your brain's learning and reward system. When your dopamine receptors get activated by something, your brain wants MORE. The original design of this was critical to our survival. If you found a bush of berries, it was paramount to want to find more of these. The problem is because tech companies understand how to activate this to maximize addiction, the dopamine reward system has been hijacked from our smartphones.

People exhaust their dopamine system with social media and apps. This leaves the average person with little to no drive to accomplish things. Their "will power" is drained because their dopamine receptors are exhausted.[202]

Every time you post something and someone interacts with it with a like, share, or comment - your brain's reward system goes off. Every time you get notifications about incoming emails, messages, or other things your brain feels, *"Hmm, I guess I'm important"*.

So most of us are trapped in these dopamine loops to various degrees. There are several things we can do to manage that.

---

[202] *Smartphones, or the greatest addiction in history of mankind.* Retrieved 2 October 2020, from https://ymedialabs.com/smartphone-addiction

Powermove: Limit Phone Usage

1 - Do not use your phone in the morning first thing when you wake up
2 - Leave your phone away from your desk while you're working
3 - Do not use your phone for a couple of hours Before bed

By doing these 3 simple things, you'll be able to enjoy your phone without completely exhausting your dopamine receptors.

BiOptimizing Your Emotional Brain

The limbic system is one of the components of our nervous system. It's considered the "emotional brain". One of the most powerful things you can do for your health is to "clean your limbic system". Why?

Many insomniacs have emotional trauma that creates painful emotional loops. These obsessive, compulsive thought patterns can make it difficult to fall asleep and lead to major health problems, which we talked about in chapter 11.

Potent Emotional Cleansers

Some of the most powerful techniques for cleaning the limbic system include:

1 - EFT, also known as tapping. Check out www.eftuniverse.com for loads of research and data.

2 - Effective Forgiveness.

   a/ First, create lists of all your fears, resentments, and other negative emotions.

   b/ Get into a relaxed, meditative state.

   c/ Replay the event and feel the emotional pain and sensation in your body.

   d/ Forgiveness Part 1 - GRATITUDE - What's The Gift of the experience?

   e/ Forgiveness Part 2 - Take responsibility for the experience.
   Take ownership of your part in that event.

   f/ Forgiveness Part 3 - Put Yourself In Their Shoes.
   Aim to understand why they did what they did.

g/ Forgiveness Part 4 - Compassionate Empathy.
Feel compassion for their shortcomings.

h/ Forgiveness Part 5 - Unconditional Love.
Aim to let go and give as much love as possible to the person.

BiOptimizing Your Work Schedule

One of the books that set us on the right track in regards to energy management is *"The Power Of Full Engagement" by Tony Schwartz and Jim Loehr."*

They were studying top tennis pros and trying to find what was their edge. Why were the top 5 better than the rest?

They analyzed everything: their swings, their serves, their cardio and they couldn't find a clear edge.

Finally, they saw that the top guys would play with their rackets in between plays. They would get their mind off the game for a few seconds. This would allow them to recover just a little bit mentally and physically in between points.

The 3 Levels of Recovery: Micro, Macro, and Meso

It's powerful to manage your energy like an athlete. Top-level athletes understand every aspect of recovery and know that it's vital for their success.

Athletes use different levels of recovery to maximize their results. They use micro recovery to keep themselves at a peak level during a workout. Athletes might take rest between sets of 15 seconds to 2 minutes.

They use macro recovery to recover from tough workouts and when they need a break. Athletes usually take 1 to 2 days off a week to allow their nervous system and muscles to recover.

They use meso recovery to cycle through various types of workouts and give their bodies a deep rest to prevent burnouts and injuries after big events and competitions. Some athletes will do completely different styles training for several months like a strength training cycle. Some athletes will take 1 to 2 weeks off, once or twice a year to allow their bodies to recover from small injuries and to replenish motivation.

How can we apply this principle in our lives to maximize productivity and manage our nervous system?

Micro-Recovery

Micro-Recovery is vital to keep mental focus strong and fresh throughout the day.

For work:

Option 1: Work 25 minutes and take 5 minutes off.
Option 2: Work 45-50 minutes and take 10-15 minutes off.
Option 3: Work 90 minutes and take 30 minutes off.

Business expert, Eben Pagan, recommends that we "change the channel" during our micro-recovery. It's powerful to CHANGE the environment.

Here are some powerful micro-recovery ideas that will change the channel:

- Going for a walk in nature
- Rebounding
- Catch some sun and a tan
- Play an instrument
- Eat
- Call a friend, a loved one, or your family
- Cuddle with your partner
- Play with your pet
- Take a nap

Macro-Recovery

We also need some days completely off to refuel the tank. We don't personally know anyone who has worked several weeks non-stop WITHOUT hitting the wall. For your macro-recovery days, aim to create YOUR PERFECT DAYS.

Perfect Days

Other than rare occasions, it's ideal for your nervous system to take one to two days off every week. Use them to spend time with friends, go on mini trips, enjoy nature, eat great food, watch movies and relax deep. Every weekend, aim to live your perfect weekend.

Meso-Recovery

Ideally, you would take a week off every 3-4 months. Having a full 9 days to recover (2 weekends plus a workweek) is usually enough to reboot the nervous system. It also does wonders for the brain and productivity.

This is often where you'll be able to get altitude on your life and business. Now that you're not caught in the trenches, you'll have the mental space to have epic visions and create new strategies. So even for the obsessed workaholic, it's a very profitable habit to take time off on a regular basis.

The Best Healing Body Work and Biohacks

Float Your Worries Away

As far as shifting the body into a parasympathetic state and allowing the nervous system to reboot, floating in a sensory deprivation tank might be the most effective modality.

A sensory deprivation tank is designed to eliminate all light and sound. The water temperature is the same as your body so you don't sense the water. And you're literally floating in a salty magnesium soup, made with Epsom salts. All your senses get a reset. You're not getting any stimuli.

There's nowhere else you get this kind of sensory reprieve. Even if you're sitting in a chair, or lying in a bed, you'll feel gravity. But when you're floating, you feel almost nothing. After a few minutes, you're not really feeling the water. You don't have light that's stimulating your brain. It's completely pitch black. There's no sound plus you're absorbing magnesium.

Acupuncture: The Power of the Needles

Acupuncture can have powerful effects on the nervous system. They can instantly shift the nervous system from sympathetic to parasympathetic.

How does it work?

Here's a theory from Dr. Ting Bao, an integrative medical oncologist at Memorial Sloan-Kettering Cancer Center in New York: *"One major hypothesis is that acupuncture works through neurohormonal pathways. Basically, you put the needle through specific points in the body and stimulate the nerve. The nerve actually sends signals to the brain, and the brain releases neural hormones such as beta-Endorphins. By doing that, the patient may feel euphoric, or happy, and this increases the pain threshold and they feel less pain."*

Get Cracked

If your spine is out of alignment, your body will be in a chronic low-level state of fight-flight-freeze. A good chiropractor will be able to take load off the nervous system.

Healing Massages

Massages can be divided into 2 categories: sympathetic or parasympathetic. If you're gritting your teeth because of the pain and intensity it's a fight-flight-freeze experience. Massage styles that emphasize intense stretching and muscular release usually fall in this category.

However, if you're drifting in and out of consciousness and passing out then it's a healing experience. Swedish massage and other types of relaxing styles fall in this category.

Other Body Work

There are too many other types of bodywork to mention in this book: Reiki, Myofascial Release, Trigger Point Therapy, Craniosacral Therapy, Kinetic Body Therapy, Polarity, Rolfing, etc... The point is, that using these can do wonders for getting your body out of the fight-flight-freeze state and into healing.

The #1 Mineral to Optimize Your Nervous System

There is 1 mineral we strongly recommend doing in high dosages: magnesium. It's saved both of us from burn out. It's healed our nervous systems more than anything else we've ever tried.

Even If You Eat or Take Magnesium (You're Almost Certainly STILL Deficient)

FACT: Over 80% of Americans are deficient in magnesium (most of the soil in the United States is lacking it). And over 99% are lacking the OPTIMAL DOSE.

Magnesium is responsible for 300-600 different biochemical reactions in the body (including metabolism). When your levels are low, you struggle with sleep, energy, metabolism, pain, and more. Worst of all, this deficiency has a very "toxic relationship" with stress.

According to Dr. Leopald Galland, M.D. — *"stress increases the amount of this nutrient we lose from our body (in urine), leading to a dangerous deficiency."*[203]

In turn, that deficiency WORSENS our response to stress. So we get stuck in a cycle of feeling stressed,

---

[203] Galland L. (1991). Magnesium, stress and neuropsychiatric disorders. *Magnesium and trace elements, 10*(2-4), 287–301.

losing more magnesium, reacting even more to stress, losing more again, and so on.

It's A Vicious Cycle...

This isn't theory: chronic deficiency of this nutrient is a bonafide epidemic.

And studies show a direct correlation between deficiency and levels of anxiety and stress.[204]
And stress ruins nearly every aspect of your health, in part, because stress increases stress hormones like cortisol, adrenaline, and noradrenaline.

In fact, a Yale study found that stress can cause abdominal fat in otherwise slender women.[205]

Why This Is the ONLY NUTRIENT That Defeats Stress at a Cellular Level

A 2010 review of natural treatments for anxiety found that magnesium could be a treatment for anxiety.[206]

More recently, a 2017 review that looked at 18 different studies found that magnesium did reduce anxiety.[207]

These studies looked at mild anxiety, anxiety during premenstrual syndrome, postpartum anxiety, and generalized anxiety.

According to this review, one of the reasons why magnesium might help reduce anxiety is that it may improve brain function.

Now, you might be thinking... *"there are a gazillion magnesium products out there, if magnesium were the solution to stress — more people would be stress-free."*

The Problem Is Two-Fold

FIRST, almost everyone is SEVERELY deficient in magnesium — even those who get the "recommended daily dose"...

---

[204] Cuciureanu, M. D., & Vink, R. (2011). Magnesium and stress. In R. Vink (Eds.) et. al., *Magnesium in the Central Nervous System*. University of Adelaide Press.

[205] Epel, E. S., McEwen, B., Seeman, T., Matthews, K., Castellazzo, G., Brownell, K. D., Bell, J., & Ickovics, J. R. (2000). Stress and body shape: stress-induced cortisol secretion is consistently greater among women with central fat. *Psychosomatic medicine, 62*(5), 623–632. https://doi.org/10.1097/00006842-200009000-00005

[206] Lakhan, S. E., & Vieira, K. F. (2010). Nutritional and herbal supplements for anxiety and anxiety-related disorders: systematic review. *Nutrition journal, 9*, 42. https://doi.org/10.1186/1475-2891-9-42

[207] Boyle, N. B., Lawton, C., & Dye, L. (2017). The Effects of Magnesium Supplementation on Subjective Anxiety and Stress-A Systematic Review. *Nutrients, 9*(5), 429. https://doi.org/10.3390/nu9050429

Because higher stress levels (common for ambitious folks like us) require much higher than RDA doses. And SECOND...

If You're *Only* Taking ONE Form of Magnesium — *YOU ARE STILL DEFICIENT*

At BiOptimizers, we're into becoming superhumans and that requires pushing the dosage to a higher level. So we did about 5 grams a day divided into 4 doses — and within a couple of months, it fixed our stress and burnout issues.

Brain came back, mood went back to normal, and performance in the gym went to another level.

Magnesium is the fourth most abundant mineral in the body and is needed for *everything*, including:

- Maintaining normal muscle and nerve function[208]
- Keeping a healthy immune system[209]
- Maintaining normal heart rhythm[210]
- Building strong bones[211]
- And lowering cortisol levels[212]

In fact, in the last study cited above — the researchers were quoted as saying, "magnesium status is highly associated with stress levels."

Magnesium has been proven to help your mitochondria generate and use ATP, the main unit of energy in the body's cells.[213] That's why another study says, "mitochondria are intracellular magnesium stores."

It's easy to see why — trying to reduce stress levels WITHOUT adequate magnesium and the full spectrum of magnesium types — is setting yourself up to fail.

---

[208] Jahnen-Dechent, W., & Ketteler, M. (2012). Magnesium basics. *Clinical kidney journal, 5*(Suppl 1), i3–i14. https://doi.org/10.1093/ndtplus/sfr163

[209] Tam, M., Gómez, S., González-Gross, M., & Marcos, A. (2003). Possible roles of magnesium on the immune system. *European journal of clinical nutrition, 57*(10), 1193–1197. https://doi.org/10.1038/sj.ejcn.1601689

[210] Magnesium helps the heart keep its mettle. Food, and maybe a multivitamin, should provide all the Mg you need. (2011). Harvard heart letter : from Harvard Medical School, 21(6), 2.

[211] Castiglioni, S., Cazzaniga, A., Albisetti, W., & Maier, J. A. (2013). Magnesium and osteoporosis: current state of knowledge and future research directions. *Nutrients, 5*(8), 3022–3033. https://doi.org/10.3390/nu5083022

[212] Cuciureanu, M. D., & Vink, R. (2011). Magnesium and stress. In R. Vink (Eds.) et. al., *Magnesium in the Central Nervous System.* University of Adelaide Press.

[213] Kubota, T., Shindo, Y., Tokuno, K., Komatsu, H., Ogawa, H., Kudo, S., Kitamura, Y., Suzuki, K., & Oka, K. (2005). Mitochondria are intracellular magnesium stores: investigation by simultaneous fluorescent imagings in PC12 cells. Biochimica et biophysica acta, 1744(1), 19–28. https://doi.org/10.1016/j.bbamcr.2004.10.013

Why Getting ALL 7 FORMS of
Magnesium Transforms Your Stress and Performance

One of the biggest misconceptions about magnesium is that you just "need more" of the mineral and you'll be healthy and optimized.

But the TRUTH is, there are many different types of magnesium — and each play a critical role in different functions in your body.

Most "healthy" people only get 1-2 forms at best (much of the population is deficient in ALL forms) — but when you get all 7 major forms of magnesium, that's when the magic happens.

We're talking about...

- Magnesium Chelate — which is especially important for muscle building, recovery, and health.[214]

- Magnesium Citrate — which helps with the effects of obesity. In fact, one study found this form was one that helped arterial stiffness in healthy overweight individuals.[215]

- Magnesium Bisglycinate — this form is most often used to help improve sleep.

- Magnesium Malate — some believe this to be the most bioavailable form (found naturally in fruits, giving them "tart taste").[216] It can help with migraines, chronic pain, and depression.

- Magnesium Aspartate — a form of the mineral that helps the connection between your brain and muscles, your cardiac rhythms, and the overall acid-alkaline balance in your body. It also can support an elevated mood.[217] It is absolutely essential in the metabolism of macronutrients, as well as the utilization of other minerals, B-complex vitamins, as well as vitamin C and vitamin E.

[214] *Chelated Magnesium Uses, Side Effects & Warnings* - Drugs.com. (2019). Retrieved 2 October 2020, from https://www.drugs.com/mtm/chelated-magnesium.html

[215] Schutten, J. C., Joris, P. J., Mensink, R. P., Danel, R. M., Goorman, F., Heiner-Fokkema, M. R., Weersma, R. K., Keyzer, C. A., de Borst, M. H., & Bakker, S. (2019). Effects of magnesium citrate, magnesium oxide and magnesium sulfate supplementation on arterial stiffness in healthy overweight individuals: a study protocol for a randomized controlled trial. *Trials, 20*(1), 295. https://doi.org/10.1186/s13063-019-3414-4

[216] Uysal, N., Kizildag, S., Yuce, Z., Guvendi, G., Kandis, S., Koc, B., Karakilic, A., Camsari, U. M., & Ates, M. (2019). Timeline (Bioavailability) of Magnesium Compounds in Hours: Which Magnesium Compound Works Best?. *Biological trace element research, 187*(1), 128–136. https://doi.org/10.1007/s12011-018-1351-9

[217] Chouinard, G., Beauclair, L., Geiser, R., & Etienne, P. (1990). A pilot study of magnesium aspartate hydrochloride (Magnesiocard) as a mood stabilizer for rapid cycling bipolar affective disorder patients. *Progress in neuro-psychopharmacology & biological psychiatry, 14*(2), 171–180. https://doi.org/10.1016/0278-5846(90)90099-3

- Magnesium Taurate — this is the form of magnesium best for your heart. One study noted: "The complex magnesium taurate may thus have considerable potential as a vascular-protective nutritional supplement." [218]

- Magnesium Orotate — While also helpful for the heart, magnesium orotate is believed to be the best form for metabolic improvements, making it a favorite for athletes wanting enhanced recovery, energy, and performance.[219]

Getting all of these forms of magnesium, in the optimum dose, upgrades virtually every function in your body.

Most Magnesium Supplements FAIL to Help You Beat Stress...

Now that you understand how critical magnesium is for everything — it might be tempting to run out to your local drug or health food store and buy some magnesium.

That would be a mistake, though — because magnesium products do nothing, for two primary reasons:

1 - They are synthetic, unnatural, and not recognized by your body and...

2 - They are NOT FULL SPECTRUM

Which means they are missing the various forms of magnesium needed to target various organs in the body and to handle all sources of stress — and boost your performance in every key area.

But there's a miracle that occurs when your body gets ALL the magnesium that it needs, in all the forms that it needs at the optimal dosage.

If You Want To Beat Stress, Get Fit, Sleep Better And Recover Faster...
You Need FULL SPECTRUM Magnesium

Whatever your diet or workout goals, magnesium can help make it work better.

However, without adequate magnesium, you're setting yourself up to FAIL.

Why? One reason is that you tend to lose a lot more water from the body in the initial state of most diets (especially lower-carb diets.)

---

[218] McCarty M. F. (1996). Complementary vascular-protective actions of magnesium and taurine: a rationale for magnesium taurate. *Medical hypotheses, 46*(2), 89–100. https://doi.org/10.1016/s0306-9877(96)90007-9
[219] Rosenfeldt F. L. (1998). Metabolic supplementation with orotic acid and magnesium orotate. Cardiovascular drugs and therapy, 12 Suppl 2, 147–152. https://doi.org/10.1023/a:1007732131887

Glycogen is stored in the body as one-part glycogen and three parts water. It means that more water is dumped through the kidneys, and since magnesium levels are controlled through the kidneys, this can then inadvertently cause a drop in serum magnesium levels.

So what's the solution? Magnesium Breakthrough.

We've created the first 7-magnesium blend solution that incorporates cofactors and monatomic minerals to maximize absorption. It's truly a game-changer.

90 Day Nervous System Rebuilding Process:

Week 1:   Start with 500 mg of Magnesium Breakthrough 3X a day.
Week 2-6:   Increase to 1,000 mg of Magnesium Breakthrough 3X a day.
Week 7-12:   Increase to 1,500 mg of Magnesium Breakthrough 3X a day.

Give it a shot. This formula is a game-changer for almost everyone who tries it.

Conclusion

The point is to make sure you're balancing and managing both sides of your nervous system. If you're a high charging person, integrate more parasympathetic in your life. If you're too calm and feel like a sloth most of the time, then integrate some fight and flight in your life. Get the adrenaline pumping a bit.

The Nervous System Cheat Sheet

	PARASYMPATHETIC: HEALING	SYMPATHETIC: FIGHT OR FLIGHT OR FREEZE
Exercise	Tai Chi Yoga	Weight Lifting Sports Running
Biohacking	Floating Meditation Eft Sleep	Cryo
Music	Classical Soundtracks	Heavy Metal Gangster Rap
Neurotransmitters	Serotonin Endorphins Oxytocin Anandamide	Adrenaline Noradrenaline Dopamine
Emotions	Gratitude Happiness Joy Peace Serenity	Fear Anger Drive/Willingness Any Emotional Reactivity
Lifestyle	Hanging With Pets Playing With Kids Making Love Walking in Nature Relaxing at the Beach	Work Intense Sex
Supplements Drinks	Reishi L-Theanine CBD/CBN/CBG Lavender Oil Ashwagandha Magnesium	Coffee Stimulants THC Nicotine
Brain Waves	Alpha Theta Delta	Beta Gamma

Chapter 15

Biological Optimizer #6: BiOptimizing Your Brain

In this chapter, you will learn:

- **How to shift the "gears" of your brain and double your productivity.**

- The secret to hacking deeper states of meditation and happiness.

- **Use your optimum breathing pattern to unlock more powerful brain performance.**

- And much more...

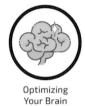

Optimizing
Your Brain

The mind shapes the body and the body shapes the mind. The good news is, by following and integrating the habits laid out in this book your brain will operate at its peak.

The great news is, you can improve your brain by training it and optimizing it with various brain techs.

Optimizing your brain is critical. According to Dr. Bravermen, author of the book "The Edge Effect", *"The difference between a resourceful mind and senility is only one hundred milliseconds of brain speed. A massive number of Americans are losing seven to ten milliseconds of brain speed per decade beginning at age forty."*

Unless you're interested in being senile, having dementia, or suffering from Alzheimer's disease, we recommend you start taking action immediately.

The Oldest Brain Optimizer

The first ever brain optimizer was meditation. Meditation allows us to control our brain waves and move into different states of consciousness.

Breathing and Meditation

When you're breathing deeply and slowly, it activates the healing part of the nervous system. If you start hyperventilating, that activates your fight or flight response and vice versa. When you're in fight, flight, or freeze, you start hyperventilating because you're trying to get more oxygen to the brain.

Breathing is the only thing that you do, both consciously and unconsciously. In other words, you can think about your breathing and change its rate. Or it happens unconsciously. And for most people, it's unconscious the majority of the time.

Focusing on your breath is one of the best ways to start meditation. As your breath slows down, your nervous system calms down. Your brain waves start slowing down. This is one of the goals of meditation.

Slow the brain waves down from beta down to alpha and then down to theta.

There are dozens if not hundreds of breathing methods. One of the best ways to start is with a simple 5-6 second inhale followed by a 5-6 second exhale. No breath holding. Nothing fancy. We did tests that measured our nervous system's response with various breathing rhythms. One thing that was fascinating is that when someone tries to hold their breath, slow it down unnaturally, or speed it up - the HRV (heart rate variability) lowered.

Doing this for 5 minutes can have a profound shift in your state of mind. Beta waves lower. Alpha waves increase. HRV goes up.

There are dozens if not hundreds of effective meditation processes. One of the most researched is gratitude. When you're feeling gratitude, you're parasympathetic. You are in a healing mode.

The key is to focus on the sensation in your body. Focusing on the feelings "love and thanks" in your heart.

The Greatest Shortcut Ever for Brain Optimization

If you're looking for a short-cut or "hack" to maximize your brain's performance, look no further. The answer is neurofeedback. We have done hundreds of hours of neurofeedback. The results have been life-changing.

- Massive gains in EQ (emotional intelligence)
- Increases in IQ
- Being able to focus for 300% longer
- Achieving Zen-like states at will
- Boosts in creativity
- Much, much more

What is neurofeedback? It is a brain measuring feedback system. You get these electrodes wired to your brain that measure the electrical activity on the surface of your brain. Then, they feed back to you what's happening in real time via audio, visual, or kinesthetic feedback.

You choose a target brain wave, for example alpha. If you're doing the right thing and alpha is increasing, you get a reward in the form of positive, reinforcing audio tones. And if you're doing the wrong thing it goes silent or quieter. Then your brain realizes, *"Whoa, that didn't work. Let me try something else."*

When you're doing the right thing, and you're getting those rewards, your brain realizes *"Oh, okay, that's what I need to do. Let me do more of that."*

Think of it kind of like a GPS. If you're driving around and you continue on the wrong street, the GPS tells you to turn around.

If you're seeking the ultimate in mental brain enhancements, look no further. If money isn't a consideration, we suggest doing one to two dedicated brain training bootcamps per year. These are serious time and money commitments. It's usually an entire week and the costs are around $15,000 USD.

Is it worth it? If you're an entrepreneur, executive, or anyone that makes a considerable amount of money using your brain - then absolutely. Let's say you're earning $250,000 a year and you improve your capacity 20%, that's an extra $50,000 a year.

Most people's brain function begins declining in their 40s and 50s. What if you could add a decade or two of prime brain function? These years could be worth millions. Learn more at www.bioptimizers.com/brainoptimizers

Shining Light Into Your Brain

One of the most promising brain optimization technologies is photobiomodulation also known as LLLT (lower level laser therapy). You blast your brain with low-level lasers that have specific frequencies.

Here are some fascinating findings on this type of therapy:

- Increases cerebral perfusion, CBF oxygen consumption, total hemoglobin, and increased oxygenated/decreased deoxygenated hemoglobin concentrations.

- Patients with dementia reported improvements in quality of life, functional abilities (i.e., decreased incontinence and increased mobility), better sleep, fewer angry outbursts, and less anxiety and wandering after the PBM treatments.[220]

- Improves Gulf War Illness symptoms, mood, cognitive domain score, pain, sleep, and fatigue.[221]

- Has positive effects on nerve cells in a range of neurological conditions, including Parkinson's Disease (PD).[222]

- Demonstrated its value as a treatment for neurological and neurodegenerative conditions, including Alzheimer's disease.[223]

---

[220] Chao L. L. (2019). Effects of Home Photobiomodulation Treatments on Cognitive and Behavioral Function, Cerebral Perfusion, and Resting-State Functional Connectivity in Patients with Dementia: A Pilot Trial. *Photobiomodulation, photomedicine, and laser surgery, 37*(3), 133–141. https://doi.org/10.1089/photob.2018.4555

[221] Chao L. L. (2019). Improvements in Gulf War Illness Symptoms After Near-Infrared Transcranial and Intranasal Photobiomodulation: Two Case Reports. *Military medicine, 184*(9-10), e568–e574. https://doi.org/10.1093/milmed/usz037

[222] *Evaluation of dose of Photobiomodulation (Light) Therapy and Physiotherapy for Improving Quality of Life Outcomes and Mobility in Parkinson's Disease (Pilot).* (Submitted 15 November 2017). ANZCTR - Registration. Retrieved 2 October 2020, from https://www.anzctr.org.au/Trial/Registration/TrialReview.aspx?id=373999&isReview=true

[223] Zomorrodi, R., Loheswaran, G., Pushparaj, A., & Lim, L. (2019). Pulsed Near Infrared Transcranial and Intranasal Photobiomodulation Significantly Modulates Neural Oscillations: a pilot exploratory study. *Scientific reports, 9*(1), 6309. https://doi.org/10.1038/s41598-019-42693-x

---

Brain Supplements

3 foundational brain supplements we believe everyone should take are:

1 - EFA/DHA blends
2 - Magnesium
3 - Lion's Mane

The brain is an organ made up of 60% fats. It stands to reason, it needs to be fed high-quality fats in the optimal quantities to operate at it's best. As a general rule of thumb, 2 grams to 10 grams a day of EFA/DHA blend is a good protocol. The benefits of taking a high-quality essential fatty acid blend are well documented. The key element for the brain is the DHA. We went in depth discussing EFA/DHA in chapter 8 previously in the book.

We already discussed the many benefits of magnesium in chapter 14.

One of the most powerful brain supplements is lion's mane. Studies have found that lion's mane mushrooms contain two special compounds that can stimulate the growth of brain cells: hericenones and erinacines.

Lion's mane mushroom extract could be extremely powerful for the nervous system. It has been shown to reduce recovery time by 23–41% when given to rats with nervous system injuries.[224]

We recommend a loading phase of 5 grams a day for 60 to 90 days and then switch to a maintenance phase of 1 to 3 grams a day.

Powermove: Get Personalized, Customized Brain Stacks

Brain chemistry is very unique from person to person. This is why we've been working for a very long time to create personalized brain optimization stacks. There is NOTHING else like this in the industry. We've partnered with who we believe is the most brilliant

man in the world of nootropics to create breakthrough brain stacks that will take your mental performance to its peak.

Visit www.bioptimizedbrain.com for more information.

---

224 Park, Y. S., Lee, H. S., Won, M. H., Lee, J. H., Lee, S. Y., & Lee, H. Y. (2002). Effect of an exo-polysaccharide from the culture broth of Hericium erinaceus on enhancement of growth and differentiation of rat adrenal nerve cells. *Cytotechnology, 39*(3), 155–162. https://doi.org/10.1023/A:1023963509393

Conclusion

One of the most obvious and painful consequences of "normal aging" is mental decline. There's no need to suffer that fate. The tools, technology, and supplements to stop and even reverse most of that are here now. The key is to start today and maintain these brain habits for the rest of your life.

Chapter 16

Biological Optimizer #7: Heliotherapy

In this chapter, you will learn:

- **Why all the "sun is bad" advice out there can hurt your health.**

- The right level of vitamin D (and sunshine) your body needs.

Heliotherapy

- **How to supplement with vitamin D when you don't have sun access.**

- And much more…

As far as ONE THING that dramatically improves all 3 sides of the BiOptimization Triangle, THE SUN is one of the biggest needle movers. You will notice massive improvements in aesthetics as the sun will boost your muscle-building capabilities (by increasing testosterone[225]) and fat-burning (by shrinking fat cells[226]). Massive improvements in health and performance become activated once your vitamin D levels are high enough.

We live in a solar system. That means that everything on this planet relies on the power of the sun, either directly or indirectly. Recently, sunshine has gotten a bad rap. It comes down to listening to your body, rather than some scientific mumbo-jumbo that sounds good but has little practical value.

Where would you rather spend a vacation? In the middle of the Arctic circle, during 24 hours of darkness at minus 40 below zero, munching on a frozen piece of seal blubber? Or would you rather be catching some soothing rays from the sun, while sitting on a tropical beach with a warm breeze blowing over ion rich oxygen, while you sip on fresh fruit juice made from lush, local organic fruits?

Most people intuitively select the latter as their circumstance of choice, as your body inherently knows what it needs… if we can just learn to start listening to it again.

Although this hasn't been proven yet, we believe there are unknown benefits and effects from getting vitamin D from the sun versus just getting them from a supplement. As with many things in health, there are far more unknowns than things we know. There are many elements we can't measure yet and we believe that this is the case with the sun.

Vitamin D deficiency is a global health problem. With all the medical advances of the century, vitamin D

225 MYERSON, A., & NEUSTADT, R. (1939). INFLUENCE OF ULTRAVIOLET IRRADIATION UPON EXCRETION OF SEX HORMONES IN THE MALE11. *Endocrinology, 25*(1), 7-12. https://doi.org/10.1210/endo-25-1-7
226 Ondrusova, K., Fatehi, M., Barr, A., Czarnecka, Z., Long, W., Suzuki, K., Campbell, S., Philippaert, K., Hubert, M., Tredget, E., Kwan, P., Touret, N., Wabitsch, M., Lee, K. Y., & Light, P. E. (2017). Subcutaneous white adipocytes express a light sensitive signaling pathway mediated via a melanopsin/TRPC channel axis. *Scientific reports, 7*(1), 16332. https://doi.org/10.1038/s41598-017-16689-4

deficiency is still epidemic. Over a billion people worldwide are vitamin D deficient or insufficient.[227]

Vitamin D, also described, as "the Sun Vitamin" is a steroid with hormone-like activity. It's more accurately a "master hormone", which means it impacts many other hormones. It regulates the functions of over 200 genes[228] and is essential for growth and development.[229]

There are two major forms of vitamin D.[230] Vitamin D2 (ergocalciferol) and vitamin D3 (cholecalciferol). Vitamin D status depends on the production of vitamin D3 in the skin under the influence of ultraviolet radiation from the sun and vitamin D intake through diet or vitamin D supplements.[231]

Usually, 50% to 90% of vitamin D is produced by sunshine exposure of skin and the remainder comes from the diet.[232] Natural diets most humans consume contain little vitamin D. Traditionally the human vitamin D system begins in the skin, not in the mouth.

However, important sources of vitamin D are egg yolk, fatty fish, fortified dairy products, and beef liver. In addition to vitamin D's well-known role in bone and calcium metabolism, vitamin D deficiency has been linked to a long list of health conditions including atherosclerosis.[233]

Vitamin D is critical to the proper functioning of the endothelial cells that line blood vessels.[234] Without sufficient levels of vitamin D, these endothelial cells become more susceptible to damage and dysfunction that ultimately can lead to the development of atherosclerosis as well as arterial calcification.[235]

[227] Holick M. F. (2017). The vitamin D deficiency pandemic: Approaches for diagnosis, treatment and prevention. *Reviews in endocrine & metabolic disorders, 18*(2), 153–165. https://doi.org/10.1007/s11154-017-9424-1

[228] Hossein-nezhad, A., Spira, A., & Holick, M. F. (2013). Influence of vitamin D status and vitamin D3 supplementation on genome wide expression of white blood cells: a randomized double-blind clinical trial. *PloS one, 8*(3), e58725. https://doi.org/10.1371/journal.pone.0058725

[229] Koo, W., & Walyat, N. (2013). Vitamin D and skeletal growth and development. *Current osteoporosis reports, 11*(3), 188–193. https://doi.org/10.1007/s11914-013-0156-1

[230] Miraglia Del Giudice, M., Indolfi, C., & Strisciuglio, C. (2018). Vitamin D: Immunomodulatory Aspects. Journal of clinical gastroenterology, 52 Suppl 1, *Proceedings from the 9th Probiotics, Prebiotics and New Foods, Nutraceuticals and Botanicals for Nutrition & Human and Microbiota Health Meeting, held in Rome, Italy from September 10 to 12, 2017*, S86–S88. https://doi.org/10.1097/MCG.0000000000001112

[231] Wacker, M., & Holick, M. F. (2013). Sunlight and Vitamin D: A global perspective for health. *Dermato-endocrinology, 5*(1), 51–108. https://doi.org/10.4161/derm.24494

[232] DeLuca H. F. (2004). Overview of general physiologic features and functions of vitamin D. *The American journal of clinical nutrition, 80*(6 Suppl), 1689S–96S. https://doi.org/10.1093/ajcn/80.6.1689S

[233] Aggarwal, R., Akhthar, T., & Jain, S. K. (2016). Coronary artery disease and its association with Vitamin D deficiency. *Journal of mid-life health, 7*(2), 56–60. https://doi.org/10.4103/0976-7800.185334

[234] Podzolkov, V. I., Pokrovskaya, A. E., & Panasenko, O. I. (2018). Vitamin D deficiency and cardiovascular pathology. *Terapevticheskii arkhiv, 90*(9), 144–150. https://doi.org/10.26442/terarkh2018909144-150

[235] Cohn, J. N., Quyyumi, A. A., Hollenberg, N. K., & Jamerson, K. A. (2004). Surrogate markers for cardiovascular disease: functional markers. *Circulation, 109*(25 Suppl 1), IV31–IV46. https://doi.org/10.1161/01.CIR.0000133442.99186.39

Vitamin D Keeps Lead in Your Pencil

Given the link between vitamin D and atherosclerosis, Italian researchers conducted a study[236] in 143 men with erectile dysfunction (ED). The men were evaluated for penile atherosclerosis by ultrasound along with blood levels for vitamin D3. Fifty men were classified as suffering from atherosclerotic ED, 28 borderline ED, and 65 non- atherosclerotic ED.

The average vitamin D level was 21.3 ng/mL and 45.9% of the men had vitamin D deficiency (<20 ng/ml). Only 20.2% had vitamin D levels greater than 30 ng/ml. The results showed that most men with ED have low vitamin D levels and those with more severe ED had significantly lower vitamin D levels than those with mild ED.

Vitamin D deficiency was also worse in those with ED due to penile atherosclerosis than in those men with ED due to other factors. These results indicate that low levels of vitamin D3 are linked to ED and indicate that vitamin D3 levels should be measured in men with ED.

Establishing optimal blood levels of D3 may lead to better endothelial function and reduce/prevent ED. In addition to ED, low vitamin D levels have been associated with reduced testosterone levels and anabolic genes.[237]

Vitamin D's Role in Muscle Building

Vitamin D is not technically a vitamin or essential dietary factor. Vitamin D is a pro-hormone produced phytochemically in the skin, and unlike traditional vitamins, Vitamin D has its own hormone receptor (VDR).

VDRs are found in at least 36 different organs in the body. To further establish this fact and to see if Vitamin D3 may actually have an anabolic effect, researchers carried out an in-vitro study using muscle cells, insulin, leucine, and Vitamin D.[238]

The focus of this study was on the mTOR anabolic signaling pathway in muscle cells. It is well known that insulin facilitates the activation of the mTOR pathway, particularly high insulin levels. Leucine is a direct activator of the mTOR pathway and in this way can "switch on" protein synthesis in muscle cells.

---

[236] Barassi, A., Pezzilli, R., Colpi, G. M., Corsi Romanelli, M. M., & Melzi d'Eril, G. V. (2014). Vitamin D and erectile dysfunction. *The journal of sexual medicine, 11*(11), 2792–2800. https://doi.org/10.1111/jsm.12661
[237] Chen, C., Zhai, H., Cheng, J., Weng, P., Chen, Y., Li, Q., Wang, C., Xia, F., Wang, N., & Lu, Y. (2019). Causal Link Between Vitamin D and Total Testosterone in Men: A Mendelian Randomization Analysis. *The Journal of clinical endocrinology and metabolism, 104*(8), 3148–3156. https://doi.org/10.1210/jc.2018-01874
[238] Salles, J., Chanet, A., Giraudet, C., Patrac, V., Pierre, P., Jourdan, M., Luiking, Y. C., Verlaan, S., Migné, C., Boirie, Y., & Walrand, S. (2013). 1,25(OH)2-vitamin D3 enhances the stimulating effect of leucine and insulin on protein synthesis rate through Akt/PKB and mTOR mediated pathways in murine C2C12 skeletal myotubes. *Molecular nutrition & food research, 57*(12), 2137–2146. https://doi.org/10.1002/mnfr.201300074

These researchers took muscle cells and exposed them to leucine and insulin, or leucine, or insulin, or Vitamin D. Results demonstrated that the addition of Vitamin D to insulin and leucine significantly enhanced the activity of the mTOR pathway and protein synthesis.

The authors concluded that Vitamin D has the potential to directly alter protein synthesis in muscle cells. Additionally, several studies have found that low vitamin D is associated with low testosterone levels.

One study found out that men with sufficient vitamin D levels had significantly higher testosterone levels and lower SHBG (sex hormone-binding globulin) count,[239] than men who had insufficient amounts of the vitamin (or hormone) in their blood serum. SHBG binds to testosterone which lowers your FREE testosterone. Free testosterone is what really matters. If you have a high level of testosterone, but your SHBG is too high, your free testosterone will be low and you won't reap the benefits.

Another study found out that when healthy male participants take 3332 IU's of vitamin D daily for a year, they end up having 25,2% more testosterone on average when compared to placebo. Getting out in the sun may be more than just relaxing, it is anabolic for anyone who wants to build muscle.[240]

The Sun Shrinks Fat Cells?

The sun is also a great aid for anyone looking to shrink fat cells. Our body has fat cells that lie just beneath the skin. When exposed to sunlight, the blue/green wavelengths can penetrate through the skin layer and reach these cells, reducing the size of lipids droplets which then get released out of the cell.

In one study, quantification of lipid droplet size found that adipocytes in the light treated group contained significantly fewer lipid droplets compared to the control (dark) group.

This means UV light from the sun has the ability to make cells in your body store less fat.

Vitamin D and the Immune System

Vitamin D is essential for a healthy immune system. Most cells of the immune system express vitamin D receptors (VDR)[241] which enable macrophages to respond to and kill bacteria and protect us from viral infections.

[239] Wehr, E., Pilz, S., Boehm, B. O., März, W., & Obermayer-Pietsch, B. (2010). Association of vitamin D status with serum androgen levels in men. *Clinical endocrinology, 73*(2), 243–248. https://doi.org/10.1111/j.1365-2265.2009.03777.x
[240] Pilz, S., Frisch, S., Koertke, H., Kuhn, J., Dreier, J., Obermayer-Pietsch, B., Wehr, E., & Zittermann, A. (2011). Effect of vitamin D supplementation on testosterone levels in men. Hormone and metabolic research = Hormon- und Stoffwechselforschung = Hormones et metabolisme, 43(3), 223–225. https://doi.org/10.1055/s-0030-1269854
[241] Bouillon, R., Carmeliet, G., Verlinden, L., van Etten, E., Verstuyf, A., Luderer, H. F., Lieben, L., Mathieu, C., & Demay, M. (2008). Vitamin D and human health: lessons from vitamin D receptor null mice. *Endocrine reviews, 29*(6), 726–776. https://doi.org/10.1210/er.2008-0004

Vitamin D also plays a role in the function of epidermal keratinocytes.[242] This is the outermost layer of the skin where keratin-producing cells protect us against microbial, viral, fungal, and parasitic invasion.

Numerous studies have found vitamin D deficiency is strongly associated with morbidity and mortality in critically ill patients from ICU.[243] [244] [245] After administration of high doses of Vitamin D3 (540,000 IU), levels increased significantly within 2 days.[246] Other outcomes include decreased hospital length of stay,[247]reduced length of ICU stay, and in severe deficiency patients, hospital mortality was significantly lower.[248]

By now, you're probably thinking you need to boost your vitamin D levels. But, what is the right dosage? And, how long should I take it for?

The fact is, there's not a definite answer since many factors will determine how your body reacts to and absorbs vitamins D. Some of these factors are:

- Age - As we age, our body loses its ability to produce and absorb vitamin D.

- Body fat - The effectiveness of vitamin D supplementation is dependent on BMI. People with obesity will need to take up to three-times higher amounts.

- Gut health - If you have an unhealthy gut then you will not be able to fully absorb nutrients including vitamin D.

- Skin pigmentation - The darker the skin color, the more melanin in the body. Melanin absorbs the UVRs from the sun preventing them from penetrating the skin and inhibiting vitamin D production. People with darker skin tones will need to be exposed to the sun for longer periods.

---

[242] Bikle D. D. (2008). Vitamin D and the immune system: role in protection against bacterial infection. *Current opinion in nephrology and hypertension, 17*(4), 348–352. https://doi.org/10.1097/MNH.0b013e3282ff64a3

[243] Braun, A., Chang, D., Mahadevappa, K., Gibbons, F. K., Liu, Y., Giovannucci, E., & Christopher, K. B. (2011). Association of low serum 25-hydroxyvitamin D levels and mortality in the critically ill. *Critical care medicine, 39*(4), 671–677. https://doi.org/10.1097/CCM.0b013e318206ccdf

[244] Venkatram, S., Chilimuri, S., Adrish, M., Salako, A., Patel, M., & Diaz-Fuentes, G. (2011). Vitamin D deficiency is associated with mortality in the medical intensive care unit. *Critical care (London, England), 15*(6), R292. https://doi.org/10.1186/cc10585

[245] Amrein, K., Amrein, S., Holl, A., Waltensdorfer, A., Pieber, T., & Dobnig, H. (2010). Vitamin D, parathyroid hormone and serum calcium levels and their association with hospital mortality in critically ill patients. *Critical Care, 14*(Suppl 1), P589. https://doi.org/10.1186/cc8821

[246] Amrein, K., Sourij, H., Wagner, G., Holl, A., Pieber, T. R., Smolle, K. H., Stojakovic, T., Schnedl, C., & Dobnig, H. (2011). Short-term effects of high-dose oral vitamin D3 in critically ill vitamin D deficient patients: a randomized, double-blind, placebo-controlled pilot study. *Critical care (London, England), 15*(2), R104. https://doi.org/10.1186/cc10120

[247] Han, J. E., Jones, J. L., Tangpricha, V., Brown, M. A., Brown, L., Hao, L., Hebbar, G., Lee, M. J., Liu, S., Ziegler, T. R., & Martin, G. S. (2016). High Dose Vitamin D Administration in Ventilated Intensive Care Unit Patients: A Pilot Double Blind Randomized Controlled Trial. *Journal of clinical & translational endocrinology, 4*, 59–65. https://doi.org/10.1016/j.jcte.2016.04.004

[248] Amrein, K., Schnedl, C., Holl, A., Riedl, R., Christopher, K. B., Pachler, C., Urbanic Purkart, T., Waltensdorfer, A., Münch, A., Warnkross, H., Stojakovic, T., Bisping, E., Toller, W., Smolle, K. H., Berghold, A., Pieber, T. R., & Dobnig, H. (2014). Effect of high-dose vitamin D3 on hospital length of stay in critically ill patients with vitamin D deficiency: the VITdAL-ICU randomized clinical trial. *JAMA, 312*(15), 1520–1530. https://doi.org/10.1001/jama.2014.13204

- Health conditions - If you have metabolic issues such as diabetes, high blood pressure, or arthritis, the amount of vitamin D your body requires will be higher.

- Genetics - There are 4 gene variants that affect how you absorb vitamin D and ultimately leads to this deficiency.

- Virus - When you're sick, the pathogens block vitamin D absorption so your body uses up its stores. If you're sick with the flu, you'll need higher amounts to replenish.

- Location - Your location determines how much sun you get. If you're in North America, you have fewer months and even hours of sunshine than people close to the equator. So if you can't get vitamin D from the sun, you'll have to take higher supplements or use tanning beds.

All that said, it could take months before vitamin D deficiency is corrected. In regards to dosage, we recommend taking 10,000 IUs per day. It may seem a very high or even toxic dose, but you would need to take this amount for an extremely long time, years, to develop any toxicity, and even then the only real risk is hypercalcemia. Which is too much calcium in the blood and that could lead to kidney stones.

Toxicity risk can be reduced by drinking plenty of water (2.5 liters of water per day), avoiding calcium supplements, and dairy products.

Powermove:
How to Maximize Vitamin D Supplementation Effects

Take vitamin D with meals containing fat to ensure maximum absorption.[249]
Some good options are oils, butter, avocados, nuts, and seeds.

Beware of Outdated Science

It is noteworthy that science has made many advancements, however, we are often manipulated by corporations who use this science to make harmful products like chemical-laden skin creams and lotions that sound good but may be detrimental.

---

[249] Kennel, K. A., Drake, M. T., & Hurley, D. L. (2010). Vitamin D deficiency in adults: when to test and how to treat. *Mayo Clinic proceedings, 85*(8), 752–758. https://doi.org/10.4065/mcp.2010.0138

Real science does not support that sunscreen reduces the incidence of cancer or has any health benefits.[250]

When it comes to sunbathing, simply use common sense and expose yourself moderately. The sun is just like any other substance. There is a deficiency zone, minimal effective dose zone, optimal dose zone, maximum dose zone, and poison zone. Should you go in the sun every day for 2 hours and roast your skin like a chicken? Of course not.

Deficiency Zone	Minimal Effective Dose	Optimal Dose Zone	Maximum Dose Zone	Poison Zone
Below 20	20 - 50	50 - 80	80-150	Over 150

What is the optimal dose zone? We think getting 15-20 minutes three to 5 times a week will do the job for most people. Just take a brief walk on a sunny day and you can instantly tell by how great you feel, that a little sunshine is good for you. Sunlight boosts serotonin levels,[251] which is important for mood.

Your skin tone will affect how much vitamin D you absorb. People with darker skin absorb less vitamin D than those with lighter skin. The darker your skin is, you'll be able to handle more sun without burning, but you'll need to spend more time to hit the optimal dose zone. Ultimately, we recommend using data (vitamin D blood test) to measure your blood levels and optimize from there.

Should you use sunscreen? Our opinion is, it depends. If you're planning on spending hours outside and you have light skin, it's wise so you don't burn. If you're only going outside for 15-20 minutes, it's not necessary.

However, do not put anything on your skin that you wouldn't want to eat. Chemicals applied to your skin are absorbed into the body. To best protect skin from sun damage is to take care of your diet and load up on fruits and vegetables high in antioxidants. If you use sunscreen, simply select organic, naturally occurring products, and avoid chemical-laden ones. Organic extra virgin coconut oil is a great example of a product that has a natural SPF and protects and nourishes skin before and after sun exposure.

Powermove: The Vitamin D Solution for Cold Long Winters

For those that live in cold or cloudy climates, sun tanning beds are an alternative way to receive life-enhancing rays. Matt was able to get his vitamin D blood levels up to 60 using tanning beds in the winter.

250 Waldman, R. A., & Grant-Kels, J. M. (2019). The role of sunscreen in the prevention of cutaneous melanoma and nonmelanoma skin cancer. *Journal of the American Academy of Dermatology, 80*(2), 574–576.e1. https://doi.org/10.1016/j.jaad.2018.06.069
251 Sansone, R. A., & Sansone, L. A. (2013). Sunshine, serotonin, and skin: a partial explanation for seasonal patterns in psychopathology?. *Innovations in clinical neuroscience, 10*(7-8), 20–24.

Conclusion

Making sure that Vitamin D levels are optimized will make a MASSIVE difference in your aesthetics, performance, and health. Use vitamin D blood tests to find exactly how much sun and supplemental vitamin D you need to be in the optimal dose zone.

Chapter 17

The Future of BiOptimization

In this chapter, you will learn:

- **3 "futuristic" approaches to superhuman biological performance and gains**

- Why working with your genes will be a game-changer redesigning your physique and health

- **New and imminent breakthroughs in testing that allow you to fix anything in your body**

- And much more...

The future of biological optimization is incredibly exciting. Knowledge, technology, and applications are growing at an exponential rate. This chapter will discuss where we're at and then share some possible applications coming in the future.

There are 3 Levels of BiOptimization:

Level 1: Bio-modulation: factors that shift and modulate the body's functions slightly.
Level 2: Bio-enhancers: externally using things to create strong effects.
Level 3: Bio-transformers: permanently changing the body's nature.

Bio-Modulation

Bio-modulation means we're doing small shifts to your body. Taking supplements like Magnesium Breakthrough help modulate or shift your body's magnesium levels.

Bio-Modulation

Positive stressors are bio-modulators. They create adaptive responses that make the body slightly stronger.

Bio-modulators include:

- Food
- Exercise
- Sunlight
- Heat: sauna
- Cold: ice baths, cold showers, and cryo
- Supplements
- Most biohacking technologies

Powermove: Biohacking Technologies

Biohacking centers are starting to emerge. Our suggestion is, go try out these amazing technologies for yourself. Equipment like: CVACs, Live02 cardio systems, red light therapies, and many of the other tech we mentioned are great bio-modulators that you can FEEL.

Bio-Enhancers

Bio-enhancers are usually exogenous (external) substances that are used to create dramatic effects. The field of bio-enhancers has exploded in the last decade or two.

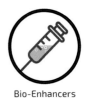

Bio-Enhancers

For example, as men get older testosterone drops (because of the 10 drivers of aging) and there is no bio-modulation strong enough to offset this drop. Yes, you can do a lot to optimize it and maintain it for a while. However, at some point the genetic programming takes hold and testosterone levels drop below the optimal zone. One of the answers is using testosterone replacement therapy. The same thing happens with stem cells and other critical substances in the body.

Bioenhancers are much more powerful and with that power comes risks. Thus they require most consideration, planning and expertise. We strongly recommend you find a qualified, knowledgeable doctor to work with when considering bio-enhancers.

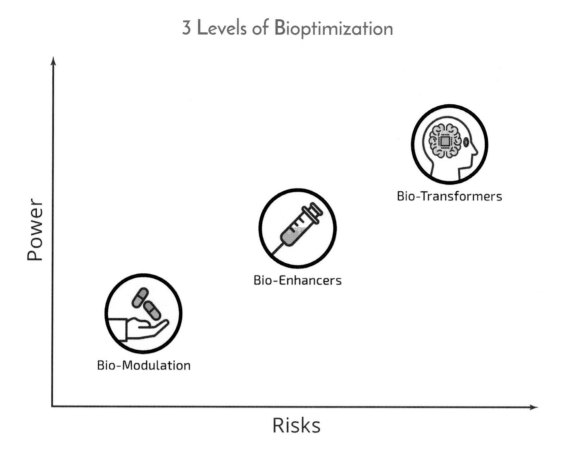

3 Levels of Bioptimization

Bio-enhancers include:

- Using exogenous hormones: testosterone, GH, progesterone, estrogen
- Stem cells including exosomes
- Peptides

With bio-enhancers, we can go beyond our genetic programming and improve healthspan massively. In other words, there is no reason to become decrepit 90-year-old men and women anymore.

Bio-Transformers

Bio-transformers use technology to create leaps in possibilities. They hold the greatest potential advancement for extending lifespan and healthspan by decades and maybe even centuries.

Bio-transformers are usually more permanent in nature and with that comes even more risks.

Bio-Transformers

A great example of bio-transformers being used today is the pacemaker. Pacemakers have saved millions of lives since 1958. Pacemakers are supplying the heart with electrical energy and helping it beat at a normal pace.

Bionic limbs are another great example that has a massive life-enhancing effect for amputees. Laser eye surgery is another great example of a bio-transformer.

We are on the cusp of mega breakthroughs in the field of bio-transformers in the next few decades.

Bio-transformers that are coming include:

- Brain to computer interfaces such as Neuralink.
- Bio-cybernetic enhancements: changing body parts with cybernetic ones.
- Genetic modifications: removing bad genes and inserting health-boosting genes

Brain to computer interfaces have tremendous implications for changing our brain's capabilities. What would the world look like if you increased the average IQ by 10 points? 30 points? 100 points? It's unimaginable. Geniuses are the ones that bring innovations that have the power to change the quality of our lives. What would the world be like if we had 100X more geniuses?

Bio-cybernetic enhancements will continue to advance. First, the focus will be to develop technologies that enhance people with severe functional issues: blindness, hearing loss, amputees, etc...

However, eventually, the market for people wanting to be truly superhuman will open up more markets. Want an exoskeleton like Wolverine? You got it!
Perhaps the most exciting and transformative field is genetic engineering.

With genetic engineering, we can edit out all genetic diseases. We can turn on genes that:

- Improve our health massively.
- Extend our lifespan by decades.
- Turn us into athletic freaks.
- Make it far easier to lose body fat.
- Make it far easier to build lean muscle mass.
- And much, much more.

Just to use one example: fat loss. We have ancient genetic wiring that helped us survive back when we were cavemen. However, this genetic wiring could be blamed for today's obesity epidemic. People are genetically wired to want to eat surpluses of sugar and fats.

The body's self-preservation genetic wiring creates many difficult challenges when it comes to losing fat. During an extended fat loss cycle, the body will:

- Lower leptin levels and slow down metabolism.
- Break down lean muscle mass for energy.

- Increase ghrelin and food cravings.
- Decrease N.E.A.T. (non-exercise activity thermogenesis), a.k.a.: move less.
- Lower hormones such as testosterone and thyroids hormones.
- And many more counter-productive reactions to our weight loss goals.

What if you could change all of that by having a 10-minute procedure? Is it the answer to obesity? Time will tell.

Evolution In Bio-Marker Tracking

As far as less radical things, one of the most exciting and powerful developments that's happening is around bio-marker tracking. The ability to track things like: sleep, glucose, steps, ketones, and much more are already available.

Within the next decade or two, we will hopefully be able to track ALL of the critical bio-markers for the fraction of today's cost.

You can easily spend $1,000 or more for comprehensive blood work and other tests. The biggest problem with current blood work is, it's a snapshot in time.

The key is CONTINUOUS DATA STREAMS.

What you measure frequently, improves rapidly.

That's the power of continuous data streams. Continuous glucose monitors (CGM) are a great example of this. Yes, it's valuable to prick your finger in the morning and see what your fasting glucose is. However, it's exponentially more powerful to see what glucose response is to all meals and activities.

When you see that your blood sugar drops by just taking a 10-minute walk, now you're motivated to do more 10-minute walks.

Imagine if you could see how your food, habits, and activities influenced your:

- Hormones: testosterone, estrogen
- Cortisol and other stress responses
- Vitamin and mineral levels
- Inflammatory markers
- And much more

Your health awareness would explode and along with it, you're motivation to change.

Conclusion

Right now, we have amazing bio-modulators and bio-enhancers available to improve our healthspan and maybe even lifespan.

With all the investments and entrepreneurial drive going into improving people's health, we can expect some breakthrough developments in biotransformation in the upcoming years and decades. Who knows? You might be amongst the first people to live to be 500 years old.

Chapter 18

The Biological Optimization Process

In this chapter, you'll learn:

- **How to know if a diet, supplement, or biohack will bring you towards Biological Optimization.**

- Our tried and true 3-step framework that has helped thousands of people achieve Biological Optimization against all odds.

- **Key biological levers to assess and test for Biological Optimization.**

- And much more...

The final chapter of this book is perhaps the most important. We are bringing together everything you've learned in this book by introducing the Biological Optimization Process.

The Biological Optimization Process

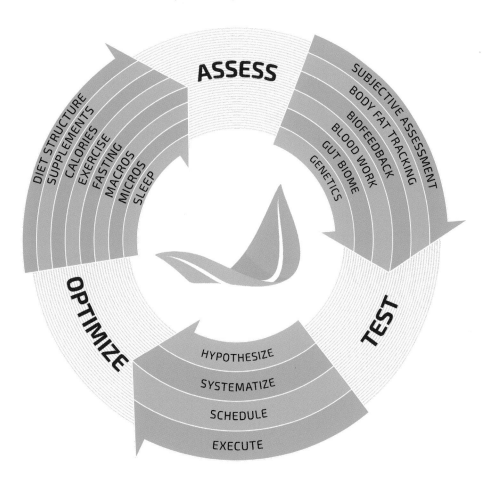

You're biologically unique, with your own sets of genes and life experience. Even the best clinical studies cannot pre-determine the right combination of diet, supplements, exercise, or biohacks that will instantly make you optimal.

Some of these add incremental gains towards your optimization goals, while others subtract. Randomly making changes without a system or understanding of biology, and you might end up going nowhere FAST (love that oxymoron!). Or you could end up in worse shape than when you started.

This chapter will teach you a scientific framework to identify things that bring you towards your goals while avoiding wasting time and money on things that set you back.

The Kaizen of Becoming a Superhuman

Rather than a "one and done" process, Biological Optimization involves iterations of Kaizen, the Japanese term for continuous improvements.

In the past 20 years, we've coached thousands of clients from all walks of life to achieve Biological Optimization against all odds. We are also standing on the shoulders of our genius mentors and coaches. We ourselves follow this Kaizen process.

Our experience and expertise have culminated in this 3-phase Kaizen framework, including:

- **Assess** - all the relevant objective and subjective data to get an accurate picture of where you are at.

- **Test** - formulate a hypothesis or a game plan before executing and testing new strategies, diets, exercise programs, and more

- **Optimize** - tweak parameters to optimize your biology with diet, supplementation, exercise, technology, and sleep

The lifelong journey of Biological Optimization never stops as you improve all three sides of the BiOptimization triangle: aesthetics, performance, and health. Going through these iterations means you will adapt and re-optimize as your health, environment, and goals evolve.

The Assessment Phase

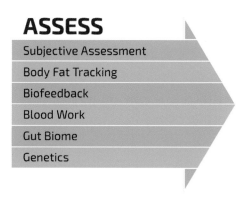

If you can't measure it, you can't improve it. To optimize, you must assess, measure, and track subjective and objective data.

Subjective Assessments

Subjective assessments are your own qualitative assessment of:

- Where you're at with respect to your challenges
- Wellbeing
- Energy levels
- Mental, cognitive, and physical performance
- Mood
- How you look in the mirror
- Appetite and cravings
- Pain and any other symptoms

Objective Assessments

Objective assessment involves measurable data of what's going on in your body, including measurable biofeedback, such as:

- Data from your Oura Ring or fitness trackers
- Lab tests
- Body composition measurements.
- And much more...

Keep in mind that wearables (such as Oura Ring or fitness tracker) don't come with standard normal values because everyone is different. To optimize your biology, first, collect and assess your data at baseline. Then, compare your progress to your baseline starting point as you go through the Biological Optimization Cycles.

Biological Levers

The following are key biological levers to assess because they provide a massive amount of useful and actionable information related to your aesthetics, health, and performance.

1 - Body Composition Tracking

Body composition tracking is a critical metric to assess where you're at both from a body fat percentage standpoint and a lean body mass perspective. DEXA (dual-energy X-ray absorptiometry) scans will also provide bone density assessment, which is important for healthspan and longevity as you get older.

If you cannot access a DEXA scan, which is the gold standard for body composition assessment, choose the next best option. You may need to use skinfold caliper, hydrostatic weighing, or Bod Pod. Body circumference measurements and pictures are also helpful pieces of data to track your progress.

We strongly caution against bioimpedance, which puts a small amount of electrical current through your body to estimate how much fat you have. These devices include the scales where you stand on two metal pads or the joysticks where you hold the metal parts. Bioimpedance doesn't measure the whole body. It can also give massive fluctuations in readings within the same day, even with high-end devices, making it a poor tool to track progress and performance.

2 - Heart Rate Variability (Oura Ring)

Heart rate variability (HRV, see Chapter 12) is a real-time measure of your stress and recovery. Persistently low HRV predicts a higher risk of sickness and deaths from all causes.[252] Therefore, to maximize healthspan and longevity, aim to maximize your HRV.

What raises HRV for one person could crash it for the next, just as one man's medicine could be another man's poison.

As an example, Matt finds that when he stays on a ketogenic diet or fasts, his HRV shot up because keto and fasting are compatible with his physiology. However, we know many people who have the opposite HRV response to keto and fasting because these dietary changes are not right for them.

---

[252] Fang, S. C., Wu, Y. L., & Tsai, P. S. (2020). Heart Rate Variability and Risk of All-Cause Death and Cardiovascular Events in Patients With Cardiovascular Disease: A Meta-Analysis of Cohort Studies. *Biological research for nursing, 22*(1), 45–56. https://doi.org/10.1177/1099800419877442

3 - Body Temperature (Oura Ring)

Body temperature is a readout of your metabolism, or how well your thyroid is working. A revved up metabolism keeps your body warm like a hot furnace.

Declining body temperature could be a sign of metabolic adaptation, which precedes a stall in your fitness results. You may need a refeed or diet break to give your body a break.

4 - Sleep Tracking

Optimal sleep is the #1 ingredient for all health goals. If you don't have your finger on the pulse of your sleep quality and quantity to optimize your sleep, you likely will waste years of your life on unrestful sleep.

Matt used to need 8 - 9 hours of sleep and was still waking up tired.

When he started tracking sleep with the Oura ring, he was shocked to learn that he was getting nonexistent deep sleep each night. After years and thousands of dollars of sleep optimization, he now gets 75 minutes - 2 hours of deep sleep nightly. Now, he only needs around 6 to 7 hours to wake up refreshed and perform optimally.

The best sleep trackers use EEG (which measures your brain's electricity). Go see the book resources for our suggestion for the best sleep trackers.

5 - Physical Performance Tracking

How you feel and how well you perform during your workouts is a crucial piece of biofeedback to your nutrification, sleep, stress, and health.

Exercise is a hormetic stimulus to elicit certain responses, such as increasing strength, muscle gain, muscle retention, or neurologic changes. To reap these benefits, you need to be able to recover from the workouts. If your performance isn't improving over time, you may need to adjust the program.

If you're in a fat loss program, one of the parameters to monitor is strength. If you're losing strength or if your reps are going down, then you're likely losing some muscle tissue. You may need a refeed, an increase in protein or amino acid intake, or ease up on the caloric deficit.

6 - Lab Tests

Men's health, performance, and aesthetics expert Dr. Paul Maximus ND routinely uses the following lab tests.

General Screening

These are common screening tests you can get from your medical doctor, including:

- *Fasting glucose* is a measure of your insulin sensitivity and ability to handle carbs.

- *Fasted insulin** will give a fuller picture of your blood sugar regulation than fasting glucose alone. For example, it is possible to have normal fasting glucose but very high insulin, which means that you are insulin resistant.

- *Cholesterol* assesses your metabolic health, risk of heart disease and Alzheimer's, and many other conditions.
- *Liver function tests* include GGT* (gamma-glutamyl transferase), other liver enzymes, and some proteins in your blood. GGT is the best indicator of health and your oxidative stress level.

- *Kidney function tests* screen for any issues with your kidneys, including diabetes and hypertension.

- *Complete Blood Count* screens for anemia, some nutrient deficiencies, blood disorders, and infections.

*In a general checkup, your doctor will typically not order GGT and fasted insulin, so you will have to specifically request them.

Spectracell Micronutrient Test

This test checks for your micronutrient status over a 3 - 6 months time window. They split your blood into 30 different sample tubes to test for micronutrients like Vitamin C, calcium, magnesium, and chromium, etc. This test also looks at your metabolism, oxidative stress, and immune response.

Protein Unstable Lesion Signature (PULS)

PULS estimates your heart attack risk by measuring the traces of proteins that leak from heart lesions in the blood vessel walls, along with HDL, inflammatory proteins, and HbA1c. Based on this, the report estimates your heart age and the likelihood of getting a heart attack in the next 5 years.

DUTCH: Dried Urine Test for Comprehensive Hormones

DUTCH provides a very illuminating snapshot of your stress response, circadian rhythm, hormone levels metabolism, and toxic hormone metabolites. It is a non-invasive urine test where you send in dried filter papers that have been saturated with your urine samples. We recommend the DUTCH Complete, which includes both adrenal and sex hormones. They also now test for neurotransmitters, vitamin, melatonin, and oxidative stress markers in your urine.

The 4-point daily cortisol pattern assesses your stress response and circadian rhythm, which could also be abnormal due to inflammation. The ratio of stress hormones to prohormones (DHEAS and pregnenolone) can tell whether your stress is stealing the resources from your sex hormone production, causing hormone imbalances.

Lastly, your toxic hormone metabolites and your hormone metabolism pattern may explain some hormonal symptoms such as hair loss, low libido, weight gain, or acne. Some toxic metabolites increase cancer risks. The DUTCH report also tells you which pathways are responsible for these hormonal issues, so you can address them naturally.

7 - Gut Biome

The 100 trillion bacteria in your large intestine work like an extra organ that masterminds all aspects of your health. A rich and diverse microbiota full of friendly species will keep you lean, healthy, happy, and resilient. Conversely, lacking a diverse microbiome and having more unfriendly strains can keep you suboptimal or sick.[253]

Tests like Viome can assess the bacteria in your gut. They also tell you which foods are best for your good bacteria, and which ones feed the bad one. Understanding your bacteria can help you optimize your diet for the optimal microbiome. The key is to eat and live right for your microbiome.

Biome Breakthrough is one of the most powerful solutions to optimize your gut health.

8 - Genetics

Your genes load the gun, while your environment pulls the trigger. Genetics is not a life sentence. Rather, you can adjust your gene function and mitigate unfavorable genetics with epigenetics.

Genetics is a vast field, and you have over 20,000 genes and numerous ways to change your epigenetics. So, we recommend empowering yourself with a nutrigenomics expert who can help you assess your genes and develop an effective epigenetic optimization protocol. See our addendum on the Jedi Council to learn about them.

---

253 Shreiner, A. B., Kao, J. Y., & Young, V. B. (2015). The gut microbiome in health and in disease. *Current opinion in gastroenterology, 31*(1), 69–75. https://doi.org/10.1097/MOG.0000000000000139

Connecting Objective and Subjective Assessments

As you become more experienced in your BiOptimization journey, you will become more in tune with your body. Your subjective assessments will dramatically improve when you connect the body's sensations to hard data.

You will notice that how you feel correlates strongly with certain objective measurements, such as:

- Feeling refreshed after a night of great quality sleep correlates with high deep sleep scores, high HRV, and low resting heart rate.

- Sensations in your body, such as feeling cold or fatigue, that indicate your body temperature dropping when you are in an aggressive caloric deficit.

- Feeling extra soreness and inflammation when your HRV is low the day after hard training.

- Having a better mood and cognitive function once your HRV improves.

- Feeling fewer cravings once your sleep and nutrition status become optimized.

Powermove: Data

Get an Oura Ring or fitness tracker and start to track your baseline data, then learn how to read and interpret the data.

Testing Phase

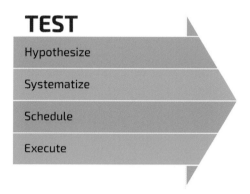

Once we have the data from the assessments, we move onto the testing phase. During this phase, we follow an n = 1 scientific game plan to test out ways to optimize your biology.

You may be self-motivated enough to coach yourself, but we recommend working with a knowledgeable coach to keep you accountable and troubleshoot as problems arise. See the Jedi council in the appendix to learn more about this. Or go to www.bioptimizers.com/coaching

Hypothesize

Hypothesizing involves formulating an educated guess about changes that will likely lead to the desired outcome. These could be the changes in your exercise, supplement stack, diet, biohacking technologies, lifestyle changes, or other health modalities. An experienced coach will hypothesize based on pre-existing science, their clinical experience, and your data from the assessment phase.

Systematize

A guaranteed way to fail is to do what you feel like doing or change your plans randomly. The lack of a system will cause confusion and prevent results. Also, trying too many changes at once, and you will not know which ones produce the results or side effects.

Systematization is all about creating a great game plan. Make sure you have a systematized exercise, nutrition, and supplementation program. Systematize whatever approach you're trying to incorporate in your Biological Optimization journey.

Schedule

Failing to plan is planning to fail. To ensure that implementation happens, you must plan it in your schedule. Scheduling is one of the most powerful ways to ensure that you stick to your plan, and thus guarantee your success!

In other words, plan and build a routine, and stick to them:

- put your workouts in your schedule
- plan your diet and prep your food for the week
- create your supplement stack on paper and stick it on your fridge door or even better preload all of your pills in a weekly pill case.

Execute

Executing the game plan is the most important part. Even a poorly executed plan is much better than the greatest plan on earth that never gets executed.

Optimization Phase

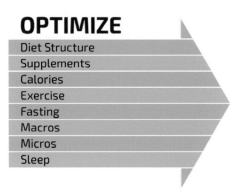

OPTIMIZE

Diet Structure
Supplements
Calories
Exercise
Fasting
Macros
Micros
Sleep

During this phase, we optimize certain parameters for the best results. The biological levers for optimization include diet structure, caloric intake, supplements, and exercise programming.

Diet Structure and Nutrition

Diet structure refers to the kind of diet you will follow. Are you going to follow a ketogenic diet, a high-carb low-fat diet, a Paleo diet, or some other type of diet?

What macronutrient composition will you follow? Typically, high protein, along with a caloric surplus, will improve muscle anabolism during a muscle-building phase. Whereas, when you are in a caloric deficit, the high protein will preserve muscle tissue.

Manipulating carbs and fats are also important to help you achieve your goals. Every diet works, including high-carb/low-fat diets and high-fat/low carb diets, as long as you are in a caloric deficit. However, the best macro for you may depend on your genetics and, to some extent, your environment, which is why we reassess.

Lastly, micronutrients, including trace minerals, vitamins, and other nutrients, are essential for your health, aesthetics, and performance. If you can't get optimal levels from your diet, then you need to supplement them.

Feeding/Fasting Window

Fasting overnight every day is important for autophagy and rejuvenation, as mentioned earlier in this book. You may find that extending the fasting window delivers more health benefits, such as fat loss, improved insulin sensitivity, and improved performance. Therefore, the fasting protocol and feeding window is another diet parameter to optimize.

Calories

Your caloric intake is another biological lever with a massive impact on the results you get, be it muscle building, fat loss, or longevity. If you want to gain muscle mass, then you need to be in a caloric surplus. If your goal is to lose body fat, you typically need to be in a caloric deficit. Lastly, if your goal is longevity, then you should be in a slight caloric deficit.

Supplements

We spent a great deal talking about supplements in this book. Supplements can have massive impacts on your results, so it is important to optimize your supplement protocol.
Some supplements are beneficial on an ongoing basis. In contrast, others may have more benefits when you start on a high dose or cycle them. Other times, you may find some supplements to do nothing or set you back. Therefore, it is essential to re-assess the impact of your supplement protocol with data.

Exercise

Exercise includes all types of movements we've covered, as well as resistance training. These have massive effects and impact on all three sides of the BiOptimization triangle: aesthetics, performance, and health goals.

Reassessment Phase (and Future Iterations)

After you have implemented the Test and Optimization phases for long enough to affect your physiology, it's time to reassess your bloodwork, body fat, biofeedback, and gut biome to see which changes are happening.

You will then learn whether your hypothesis were true, or whether you need to refine them further or develop alternate ones. Then you will follow the same process to test and optimize.

One of our core values at BiOptimizers is to test, learn, grow, and evolve. That core value is the process that drives the Biological Optimization process. We're testing things, we're learning, we're growing from them, and eventually, we evolve.

Successful BiOptimization requires knowledge, wisdom, discipline, and, often, problem-solving from experienced experts. Studies have also shown that accountability makes people 65% more likely to adhere and follow-through with whatever diet and strategy they're using.[254]

This is why we are offering our coaching to those who are serious about their journey into Biological Optimization. Visit www.bioptimizers.com/coaching for more information.

[254] Lemstra, M., Bird, Y., Nwankwo, C., Rogers, M., & Moraros, J. (2016). Weight loss intervention adherence and factors promoting adherence: a meta-analysis. *Patient preference and adherence, 10,* 1547–1559. https://doi.org/10.2147/PPA.S103649

Chapter 19

Living The BiOptimization Lifestyle

In this chapter, you will learn:

- **How to pinpoint the right diet for your body (most people get this wrong).**

- The "golden rules" that guarantee a leaner, sexier body (man or woman).

- **The most important decision you'll ever make for your biological optimization goals.**

- And much more...

Perhaps the most important "Powermove" we can share with you is: it's all about turning information into a lifestyle that you enjoy. It's about LOVING the journey. It's easy to keep going and take action when you're enjoying what you do and loving the process.

The Nutritional Lifestyle You Love

Here's what might sound like a shocking statement to many: ALL DIETS WORK.

That's right, every diet WORKS. Are there certain diets that work better than others for certain things and for certain people? YES.

However, the best diet for YOU is the one you can follow. If you don't enjoy eating meat, then keto probably isn't for you.

If you don't enjoy eating vegetables, then maybe being a vegetarian isn't for you.

Get stressed out while fasting? Then, doing an intermittent fasting lifestyle probably isn't for you.

If you have an iron will and are a disciplined person, then maybe you're someone that can follow a hyper-regimented bodybuilding-style diet.

In our upcoming nutrition book, we will go in depth and cover virtually every diet and discuss the pros and cons and help you create the best diet for YOU. For now, just follow whatever nutritional philosophy you resonate with.

The Fitness Program You Love

We only have 2 rules when it comes to fitness:

1 - Move (daily ideally).
2 - Lift heavy things (at least 3X a week ideally).

It doesn't matter what the type of movement that you enjoy to do whether it's:

- Running
- Yoga
- Biking
- Swimming
- Playing tennis
- Martial arts
- Basketball
- Walking

The benefits of MOVEMENT are the same. The KEY is making it a daily or weekly habit and PROTECTING that habit. Momentum is a very hard thing to build. Once you have built a habit, do everything in your power to keep that momentum alive.

So many times, we would get clients that would say "Yeah, I used to do _____ 10 years ago." The benefits of exercise are short-lived. What we did even a week ago, barely has any effect on us today. We must keep moving if we want the benefits.

As far as resistance training, you don't need to strive to become a muscular bodybuilder. The minimum effective dose for weight lifting is 3X a week. Three, well-structured 30-minute workouts with heavy resistance are enough to get the majority of the health benefits. You won't become Mr. or Mrs. Olympia, but you will be a much healthier person and you will experience amazing benefits.

Incorporating Powermoves Into Your Life

Every Powermove in this book has an impact on your health. Do you need to do every single one? Of course not.

Our suggestion is, start with a few simple things that speak to you and incorporate them into your life. Then, keep adding more, one at a time.

When someone who isn't into biological optimization looks at our lifestyles and habits, they usually think *"These guys are a little crazy and extreme."* To us, THIS IS NORMAL. We've been building and stacking these health habits for decades. We didn't go from couch potatoes to who we are today overnight.

Coaching and Guidance

One of the most powerful things you can do to improve your results is to get coaching.

A good coach brings:

- Motivation
- Accountability
- Guidance
- Problem-solving
- Expert tips
- And so much more

This is why we are offering coaching services to those who are serious about their journey into biological optimization. You can go to www.bioptimizers.com/coaching for more information.

We're excited to return to our roots and help YOU become the superhuman version of yourself.

The Unbreakable Commitment

We believe that one of the biggest differences between people who are living healthy lifestyles vs. people who struggle to follow healthy lifestyles is: **The Unbreakable Commitment**.

The Unbreakable Commitment is THE DECISION that you will pursue health forever. No matter what. It's a part of your life.

Goals are powerful, but The Unbreakable Commitment is 100X more powerful than that. As trainers, we would get clients that would come in with short-term goals, achieve them, and then lose motivation and go back to their old habits.

Someone who has made THE DECISION to pursue and develop health for the rest of their lives doesn't stop. When Matt got shot a few years ago, he was in the gym training with a cast. When Wade travels and is under extreme conditions, he still MAKES time to go to the gym.

Will we waver in our motivation? Of course, we're human. Will we drift away from our ideal standards at times? Of course, we're human. However, once you make The Unbreakable Commitment -- you will always course correct and get back on track. Your internal GPS is telling you to turn around.

NOW is the time. Right here. Right now. Make The Unbreakable Commitment to yourself that you will pursue biological optimization for as long as your heart beats.

APPENDIX A

Stacks and Protocols:
Creating Your Personal BiOptimization Blueprint

The appendix has various protocols and stacks that we use with our clients to help optimize and maximize their results. Choose the one that will help you get to your goals faster.

Rebuilding Your Intestinal Health Protocol

If you're having digestive issues, we suggest doing a full 90-day digestive health reboot.

In the first 30 days, your primary focus is going to be putting enzymes, probiotics, and biofilm builders into your system to get your digestive system operating efficiently.

Switching over to more whole foods products is encouraged. You may consider adding Protein Breakthrough into the diet, so you can get your body used to experiencing whole foods.

For the next 90 days, we'll be aiming to nutrify the body by giving the body the nutrients and bio-workers (enzymes and probiotics) it needs.

You'll also be adding vitamins and minerals to your regimen because they're going to enhance virtually every single cellular function and cellular communication.

What a lot of people find is after they've gone through this 90-day cycle is, they require less food in order to achieve their physical goals. And anytime you use less food, you put less strain on your body's metabolism. Most people notice how this reduces morning brain fog and the amount of sleep required to feel rejuvenated. And they will experience a new level of energy and drive throughout the day.

Upon awakening:

- 5 capsule of MassZymes
- 3 capsules of P3-OM

With breakfast (take even if you're fasting):

- 1 scoop of Biome Breakthrough (great in shakes, teas, and coffees)
- 10 drops of Primergen-V & 10 drops of Primergen-M (great in shakes, teas, and coffees)
- 3 capsule of MassZymes
- 2 capsule of P3OM

With each meal:

- 5 capsules of MassZymes
- 3 P3-OM
- 2 HCL Breakthrough

Early afternoon:

- 10 drops of Primergen-V & 10 drops of Primergen-M

Before bed:

- 5 P3-OM
- 5 MassZymes

Other tips to optimize your digestive health:

1 - Do a Viome test to see what types of foods you should focus on and which foods to minimize based on your gut health.

2 - Do a Cyrex test to see what types of foods you should avoid.

3 - Do blood tests to monitor the various blood markers to see anything should be adjusted.

The Optimal Digestive Health Stack

This is the stack we suggest for people who have good digestion but want to optimize their absorption of nutrients from their food. It delivers maximum digestive conversion and assimilation of nutrients. You'll have the right blend of enzymes, HCL, and proteolytic probiotics to breakdown virtually any kind of food you eat.

Upon awakening and before bed on empty stomach:

- 5 MassZymes
- 3 P3-OM

With each meal consume:

- 5 MassZymes
- 3 P3-OM
- 2 HCL Breakthrough

The Muscle Building Stack

This is the stack for people who want to maximize their lean muscle gains. We're increasing the MassZymes dosage to get more amino acid breakdown. This is important especially as you increase your protein intake.

Upon awakening and before bed on empty stomach:

- 5 MassZymes
- 3 P3-OM

With each meal consume:

- 10 MassZymes
- 3 P3-OM
- 2 HCL Breakthrough

Other tips to maximize your muscle gains:

1 - Consume 0.7 to 1 gram of protein a day per pound of body weight, spread out over 4-6 meals. Add 1 gram of HMB or 5 grams of leucine with the meal to maximize the mTOR response.

2 - Drink this intra-workout shake to maximize gains: Blend 2 capsules of MassZymes with your protein shake and sip while you're exercising. Add 7 drops of Primergen-V and 7 drops of Primergen-M to boost absorption even more.

3 - Focus on maximizing your deep sleep. Optimizing sleep quality is one of the most important factors. Implement every possible sleep optimizer you can afford from the sleep chapter.

4 - Learn proper exercise performance.

5 - Get out of sympathetic mode as fast as possible after your workouts.

6 - Focus on doing heavy compound movements like squats, deadlifts, dips, bench press, shoulder presses, barbell curls, etc...

7 - Change your program every 12 weeks. 12 weeks is enough time to maximize the gains from a program. After 12 weeks, your body will be adapted.

8 - Train hard, train smart. You should be close to failure on most sets. However, listen to your body and respect it if your nervous system is being overtaxed.

9 - Implementing the tips from the nervous system chapter are powerful answers to this.

The Vacation, Holiday, Party, and Cheat Day Stack

This is the stack for people who want to minimize and eliminate "damage" when they go off their diets and enjoy their favorite comfort foods and cheat meals (like SideCar donuts and Cronuts). Food is one of the joys of life and with the right tools you can enjoy all of your favorite foods and get away with it!

First, Gluten Guardian breaks down gluten and casein (from dairy) into usable amino acids. This will minimize bloating, gas, and inflammation.

As far as traveling, here's how to avoid diarrhea, food poisoning, and other problems. P3OM protects you against foreign bacteria. As far as we know, it's undefeated against food poisoning. HCL helps protect you against parasites and other invaders.

With each meal consume (if your meal is over 2,000 calories, double dose):

- 5 Gluten Guardians
- 3 P3-OM
- 3 HCL

Other tips to minimize fat gain during high-calorie meals:

1 - Do a bodybuilding style workout to use the extra calories to gain muscle. This burns far more calories than cardio. You're taking advantage of the anabolic effect of the calorie surplus. Building lean muscle mass burns a tremendous amount of energy.

2 - Do intermittent fasting for the first part of the day. By compressing your eating window, you'll eat less overall calories.

3 - Do a 2-3 day fast right after your vacation to burn off any extra fat gain.

4 - Take Berberine and other insulin sensitizers.

5 - Walk for 10 mins after each meal.

BulletProof/Keto/Paleo Diet Stack:
For Maximum Fat Breakdown and Utilization

This is the stack for people following ketogenic diets, bulletproof diets, paleo, and other high-fat diets. The idea is let's break down more of the fats that you eat into usable fatty acids. Let's transport more of them into your liver and mitochondria. Let's ramp up the liver and mitochondria's fatty acid oxidation. That's what kApex does.

For all-day energy, upon awakening:

- Consume 3-5 kApex (1 capsule per 50 lbs of body weight)

With each meal consume:

- 1 kApex (don't take after 5 pm)
- 2 P3-OM
- 1 HCL Breakthrough

Other tips to maximize your results on a ketogenic diet:

1 - Eat the highest quality fats possible. We covered this in chapter 8.

2 - Eat real foods. Minimize processed foods.

3 - Minimize A1 protein by avoiding dairy from cows. Consume dairy from other animals: sheep, goat, bison, etc...

4 - Hire a nutrigenomic expert to see if keto is the right diet for you as well as figure out your mutations. This can help you optimize your diet to the next level.

5 - Do the Viome test to see which meats, fish, nuts, and vegetables you should eat more of and which ones you should minimize.

6 - Do Cyrex to find any food sensitivities and allergies. Cut all of those foods from your diet.

7 - Experiment with a carnivore diet to see if it works well for you.

8 - Do blood tests every 3 months to monitor key health markers. Make adjustments if necessary and re-test your blood until your levels are optimal.

9 - Consume a lot of high-quality salt such as Himalayan to make sure you're sodium and mineral levels are high enough.

90 Day Total Gut Cleanse Stack:
Clean and Detox Your Intestinal Tract of Parasites and Bad Bacteria and Rebuild Your Gut Biome

For 90 days, with each meal:

- 2 Herbal Parasite Cleanse capsules (to fight parasites)
- 1 HCL Breakthrough capsules (to fight parasites)
- 2 P3OM capsules

Once a day, use one scoop of Biome Breakthrough, which has been shown in the lab tests to help defeat what is called gram-negative bacteria. It is also incredibly effective at building biofilm, in other words, it's critical to build a healthy gut lining with good bacteria.

The Brain Boosting Energy Stack:
Boost Your Brain's Energy and Mitochondria

Upon awakening:

- 3-5 kApex (1 per 50 lbs of body weight)
- 2 CogniBiotics
- 7 drops of Primergen-V (can blend with tea, coffee, water, or shake)
- 7 drops of Primergen-M (can blend with tea, coffee, water, or shake)

With lunch:

- 1-2 kApex
- 7 drops of Primergen-V (can blend with tea, coffee, water, or shake)
- 7 drops of Primergen-M (can blend with tea, coffee, water, or shake)

Fat Loss Stack:
Helps Maximize Fat Loss

Upon awakening:

- 4-6 kApex
- 10 P3-OM

With each meal:

- 1-2 kApex(don't take after 5 pm)
- 3 P3-OM
- 2 HCL Breakthrough

Before bed:

- 5 P3-OM

Fat loss tips:

1 - Find a way of lowering calories that works for you psychologically. Some people enjoy eating multiple times a day with lower calorie meals. Some people prefer eating fewer meals but eating more for each meal. For those people, intermittent fasting (IF) is a great option.

2 - Find ways of managing hunger. Some options include adding more high-protein/low-calorie foods, high-fiber/low-calorie foods (such as vegetables), or incorporating (IF), which after a few days of not eating a meal, shifts the ghrelin response (the hunger hormone) for that meal.

3 - Do two-day, high-carb refeeds at least every 2 weeks in order to help prevent metabolic adaptation. Aim to eat about 15-25% more calories above maintenance on those two days.

4 - Do diet breaks (an entire week of eating at maintenance) every 2-4 weeks in order to prevent metabolic adaptation.

5 - Slowly ramp up your cardio activity over time. Walking is probably the best for most people. Do not overdo cardio because it will speed up metabolic adaptation.

6 - Change your weight training workout every 8 weeks in order to activate more adaptation responses.

7 - Focus on optimizing your sleep. It will amplify the results of your program.

8 - Aim for 1 gram of protein per pound of bodyweight. Protein has been shown to be ideal for preventing the breakdown of muscle tissue during weight loss programs.

9 - Drink 3-5 liters of good water a day to help the body's organs (especially the liver) work optimally.

10 - Consider adding cold thermogenesis as another way to burn calories. This includes cold baths, ice vests, or cryotherapy.

The Ultimate Biological Optimization Protocol

This is the protocol that Matt and Wade use to stay optimized on all levels. This is for people that are absolutely committed to maximizing their BiOptimization Triangle. Here's the protocol:

Upon awakening:

- 4-6 kApex
- 1 capsule of Magnesium Breakthrough
- 5 capsule of MassZymes
- 5 capsules of P3-OM
- 2-4 capsules of Cognibiotics

For breakfast:

- 1 scoop of Biome Breakthrough (great in shakes, teas, and coffees). If you're fasting, save it for your eating window.
- 10 drops of Primergen-V & 10 drops of Primergen-M (great in shakes, teas, and coffees)
- 1-2 scoops of Protein Breakthrough
- 1 capsule of MassZymes
- 1 capsule of P3OM

With each meal:

- 5 capsules of MassZymes
- 3 P3-OM
- 2 HCL Breakthrough
- 1 Magnesium Breakthrough

Early afternoon:

- 10 drops of Primergen-V & 10 drops of Primergen-M
- 1-2 kApex

Post-workout shake:

- 2 scoops of Protein Breakthrough
- 2 MassZymes (mixed in the shake)
- 1 P3OM (mixed in the shake)
- 7 drops of Primergen-V and 7 drops of Primergen-M
- 2 cups of your favorite nut milk or coconut water
- 1 cup of frozen berries
- Optional: 1 scoop of Biome Breakthrough

Before bed:

- 3 Magnesium Breakthroughs
- 5 P3-OM
- 5 MassZymes

Assembling Your Jedi Council

"If you want to get the results you've never had, you must be willing to do something you've never done."
~Thomas Jefferson

In this chapter, you will learn:

- **How coaches and health advisors can shorten your path to success by months or even decades.**

- Understanding the roles of each type of health expert in your Jedi council.

- **How to choose your coaches and reap the most benefits from each of them.**

- And much more...

If you've ever watched the Star Wars series, then you've seen the Jedi Council in the movies. It's a group of wise creatures that come together and help solve the problems of the universe. This chapter is about recreating that for yourself to help you succeed with your biological optimization objectives.

If you're reading this, we believe you desire profound results with your health, aesthetics, and performance. But by this point in the book, you're probably ready for action and eager to know what to do next.

The Most Powerful Question: Who's Next?

Nowadays, the Internet is littered with health information, the majority of which is irrelevant for you. There are limitless ways to diet, supplements to take, and health hacks to try.

The most powerful question is not "What's next?", it's usually "Who's Next?" meaning that finding someone who has the information is usually more powerful and leads to greater success than "What's Next?"

There's no shortage of information. What you need isn't more information, it's wisdom. Wisdom comes from knowing which tactic and strategy to apply to each situation. A good coach, "The Who", will help you focus on the right things at the right time.

There is so much to know about the human body and health optimization that it's impossible for one person to master it all. And simply going to school is not enough, you need years or decades of hands-on experience to master each field of health.

To achieve optimal health, performance, and aesthetics, you're going to need multiple Jedis in your Jedi Council. Each of them plays an important role depending on your situation and what your goals are.

This section will help you understand the strengths and limitations of each profession so that you can make the most of working with them and give you the knowledge you need to build your Jedi Council.

You could even be an expert in the subject, like how we studied kinesiology and exercise physiology in school and trained thousands of clients. But being knowledgeable is different from being wise or being able to coordinate different pieces of information into a personalized strategy that is optimal for you.

You may think that it's possible to research anything on the internet nowadays, which is true. But this is also why 97% of dieters suffer lifetimes of yoyo dieting only to end up heavier and in worse health than when they started.[255]

The Tale of Two Bodybuilders

The Power of Personalized Coaching by Wade Lightheart

I spent the first ten years of my bodybuilding career as a "textbook" expert. I studied exercise physiology in university and read many bodybuilding books, muscle magazines, and Arnold Schwarzenegger's Encyclopedia of Training.

But after 4 years of University, I walked out with a lot of uncoordinated information. And even more importantly, I didn't get any professional feedback on what I was doing wrong and how I could improve. There's a major difference between knowledge and wisdom.

My own self-will and self-education were enough to help me win the Provincial Championship in Canada. But when I reached the National Level stage, it was obvious to me that I was not at the National caliber.

I found that the most successful competitors were all referring to a bodybuilding coach named Scott Abel. Their physiques were clearly superior to others at competitions.

That led me to reach out to Scott Abel and started working with him. In his first letter, he said:

"Your training is amateurish. Your diet doesn't do your body justice. And your performance enhancement stack is a joke!"

His words, not mine. But it excited me because I knew then that there was a lot more potential I could achieve with my results.

Over the course of the next 9 months, I made more progress than in the 10 years prior.

---

[255] Brown, H. (2015). *Planning to Go on a Diet? One Word of Advice: Don't.*. Slate Magazine. Retrieved 2 October 2020, from https://slate.com/technology/2015/03/diets-do-not-work-the-thin-evidence-that-losing-weight-makes-you-healthier.html.

It dawned on me that my ego blocked my progress for 10 years! My ego believed I could learn everything without a coach. I studied exercise physiology in university from professors. I thought I had all the answers from books and magazines.

Maybe you're thinking you've got all the knowledge you need from YouTube, social media, and podcasts? The difference between professional coaching and self-guided coaching is night and day. The key is the nuances that come from decades of experience compressed into wisdom.

The personalized guidance from a great coach can shortcut anyone's journey to excellence by years and decades. In fact, I think it's impossible to reach your full potential in anything without coaching and mentors.

Looking back, if I had Scott in the beginning, I might have been able to achieve 11 years of progress in 3 to 4 years. And my career trajectory would have been very different had I gone that route.

With Scott's guidance, I became National Champion as a natural bodybuilder and accomplished my dream of going to the Mr. Universe in India.

Since then, I've adopted this approach in all areas of my life, and it has provided me with numerous shortcuts and accelerations to success.

How I Blew a Year of My Life and Crushed My Dreams in 14 Weeks
By Matt Gallant

I got bit by the bodybuilding bug at 16 years old when I went to the beach one day and saw 2 professional bodybuilders. I was blown away and subsequently became totally obsessed with muscle growth. I started training twice a day. I went from 145 lbs to 235 lbs in 3 years, NATURALLY. I decided I wanted to compete, starting with a fair amount of muscle mass and quite a bit of fat mass to lose.

I thought I could figure it out on my own with no coach, so I started dieting and cutting calories. The first 25 lbs went smoothly and I was really happy with the results.

But then the results started slowing down because of metabolic adaptation... I made the same mistake many dieters do:

1) I decreased calories.
2) Increased exercise.

Yup, I decided to go crazy by doing 2 weight workouts a day and 90 minutes of cardio. I was working out for 3.5 hours every day.

Desperate for progress, I eventually cut my calories down to 600 calories/day. I remember I was only eating 2 ground beef patties a day because I was doing keto. I had no bowel movements for 3 weeks.

I ended up losing 64 lbs in about 14 weeks. In the process, I destroyed about 20 lbs of lean body mass, which meant I lost about a year of progress.

The worst part was, I wasn't in bodybuilding shape at all on competition day. I was gutted, having lost a year of bodybuilding progress and feeling embarrassed about how I looked. The results were just disastrous because I was trying to do it myself. I just went to my girlfriend's place and cried. That night, I went to the bar, I drank 20 shooters and they had to carry me out of there.

That was the end of my bodybuilding journey. I quit because the whole experience was a nightmare. This is a common experience for many dieters. They end up feeling depleted, deflated, and give up.

If I had the right guidance and the right coaching, I would have done everything far more intelligently. As a result, I would have kept more muscle mass and showed up to the competition in shape and possibly continued competing.

How to Fast-Track Your Biological Optimization Success

None of our education, book studying, or internet reading taught us anything about our own mental biases, unconscious bad habits and that held us back for years. By the time we realized our mistakes, we had lost time, health, and money that we couldn't get back.

The Internet will not tell you that your training is amateurish, your diet doesn't do your body justice, or that your supplement stacks make no sense.

If it does, you'd be hearing from armchair experts who may not have even achieved the same results for themselves or thousands of clients. People can't give you what they don't have.

If you want the shortest path to lasting results you've never got, seek out the experts who have cracked the code or are at the bleeding edge of the results you desire. Their wisdom and insights could be lightyears ahead of anything that's ever been published in books, blogs, or taught in schools.

Imagine the results you could achieve...

If your success and career rely on your cognitive power, how much more money will you make if you could improve your cognitive power by 20%?

If you could keep your mental and health prime for decades more than with the right guidance, you could make a massive amount more in income over your lifetime.

If you've worked your whole career and are in your 50s and 60s, now is the time to focus the energy and resources you have to improve your quality of life for decades to come. You will also have more energy to play with your grandkids and enjoy life. This will be the most prudent investment to build your healthspan and maximize your lifespan.

3 Ways a Jedi Council Will Accelerate Your Success and Save You from Costly Mistakes

1 - Bringing Data to Life

You can't improve what you don't measure, so the best place to start from is your data. In Chapter 19, we will cover all the different biofeedback readouts that you should be aware of and test regularly.

There's the "input" data, such as how you live, eat, exercise, and think. Then, there's the "output" data, as in your biofeedback readouts, how happy you are, and how you feel and perform.

But you're not a number or a spreadsheet—every piece of data needs physiological and clinical context to bring them to life and turn them into useful information.

The data will also illuminate the root causes if there are any invisible factors keeping you from optimal health, aesthetics, and performance. Therefore, it is important to start with the data.

If you're inexperienced, it's really easy to skew the data interpretation one way or the other.

For example, our friend Ben Greenfield, a professional extreme sports athlete, possesses the FTO gene version that predicts obesity on saturated fat. By anybody's standards, he's ripped.

Ben went through a period of a strict high saturated fat diet as he trained for Ironman. Surprisingly, he didn't gain any weight and even had trouble keeping the weight on. Also, his blood markers remained optimal throughout those years.[256]

The opposite results will likely happen for a middle-aged man who has the exact same genotype but with belly fat and insulin resistance.

The best coaches can bring the data to life—they can help you make sense of it all given your goals, the context, and help you develop a plan based on your data.

Your input and output data can also show your strengths, weaknesses, opportunities, and threats. These could be your psychological, physiological, emotional, or behavioral limitations. A great health coach will play up your strengths and help you address your weaknesses, or stop a disease decades before they become a diagnosis.

---

[256] *[Transcript] - Why Your DNA Is Worthless (& What You Need To Focus On Instead). -* Ben Greenfield Fitness - Diet, Fat Loss and Performance Advice. Ben Greenfield Fitness - Diet, Fat Loss and Performance Advice. Retrieved 2 October 2020, from https://bengreenfieldfitness.com/transcripts/transcript-wild-health/.

---

2 - Personalization, Practicality, and Periodization

The health field is so vast that it is impossible for one person to know everything there is to know. The rapid growth of the internet can also further add to the confusion. Every 2 - 3 years, humans create 10x the amount of digital data generated.[257]

The more vast the internet gets, the better the marketers become at catching your attention and making their solution look like the ultimate solution.

The key to success is to ignore the noise and be laser-focused on what best applies to you right now, based on your health, performance, aesthetics goals.

Often, it's also not practical to maximize all three of them at the same time. Most people have different seasons in their lives where they focus on distinct goals while compromising others. For example, if you are cutting for a bodybuilding show, you are going to compromise your health and sometimes performance.

In fitness, we use "periodization", where we break our training down into phases. For example, we might start off a client with a few months of building form and strength before entering a muscle-building phase.

Periodization also applies to health optimization and practically any other areas of your life. For example, you may have a phase where you want to go from borderline sick to optimal, then work on optimizing mental performance. You may have a phase where you build up your wealth and skills before a phase where you focus on parenting.

Each phase has a different key focus and protocols. The key is to build a strong foundation.

Here's a great rule of thumb to remember: it takes 20% of the energy to maintain a level than it takes to reach a new one. For example, if your goal is to lose 50 lbs of body fat, that requires a high level of focus, strategy, and discipline for an extended period of time. However, once you reach your goal, maintaining your body fat and body weight still requires vigilance but it's 20% of the energy, time, and focus.

You may also have unforeseen challenges that come up, such as injuries or life events, that demand your attention. Your coach can help you adapt your program or pivot to a new phase to address those challenges.

A great Jedi master will help you periodize your health protocols based on practicality and personalization. When you transition into your next phase, you may also find it beneficial to move onto a Jedi coach and mentor who's more knowledgeable about your new phase.

---

[257] *How Much Data is Created on the Internet Each Day?* Micro Focus Blog. (2019). Retrieved 2 October 2020, from https://blog.microfocus.com/how-much-data-is-created-on-the-internet-each-day/.

3 - Accountability and Feedback

Accountability has been the biggest driver of success in our lives. There were times where we had coaches, and times where we didn't. And when we had coaches, we were far more successful.

Optimizing your diet and health is simple, but it's far from easy because change is difficult. 100% of the population know that they need to adhere to a caloric deficit to lose weight, but less than 35% of them successfully lose weight.[258]

There is a major difference between knowledge and successful implementation.

The only magic the successful 35% have found is a way of eating and exercise that works for them. Psychologically, they developed mindsets and habits that help them be consistent and focused. They know how to troubleshoot challenges rather than quit when things don't go according to plan. Most importantly, they didn't do it alone.

In a systematic review of 27 weight-loss trials, supervised programs that held participants accountable had 65% higher adherence rates than those without supervision.[259]

A weight-loss trial from the University of Texas Houston examined the impact of coaching and Fitbit technologies on weight loss programs in 500 obese patients. They found that supportive accountability measures were significantly higher in groups with a coach and FitBit monitoring compared with either FitBit alone or self-monitoring at home. These accountability measures correlated with the percentage of successful weight change.[260]

When you know that your coach is going to look at your weight and body fat measurements in a week's time, you're much less likely to go for the ice cream.

Are You Getting in Your Own Way?

Most people have unconscious biases and resistances that keep them from achieving their full potential.

For us, it was our egos. Some people self-sabotage because they're afraid of their success or have internal stories that keep them from succeeding. Your Jedi master should be able to pick this up, challenge you on it, and help you get past this block.

---

[258] Brown H. Planning to Go on a Diet? One Word of Advice: Don't. [cited 23 Sep 2020]. Available: https://slate.com/technology/2015/03/diets-do-not-work-the-thin-evidence-that-losing-weight-makes-you-healthier.html

[259] Lemstra, M., Bird, Y., Nwankwo, C., Rogers, M., & Moraros, J. (2016). Weight loss intervention adherence and factors promoting adherence: a meta-analysis. *Patient preference and adherence, 10*, 1547–1559. https://doi.org/10.2147/PPA.S103649

[260] Chhabria, K., Ross, K. M., Sacco, S. J., & Leahey, T. M. (2020). The Assessment of Supportive Accountability in Adults Seeking Obesity Treatment: Psychometric Validation Study. *Journal of medical Internet research, 22*(7), e17967. https://doi.org/10.2196/17967

There are physiological challenges that must be addressed. As an example, when it comes to weight loss our bodies have evolved over billions of years to prioritize survival. It has many survival mechanisms that can sabotage your weight loss success. This topic deserves a book of its own and it's one of the main things we focus on with our weight loss coaching clients.

Pivoting and Troubleshooting

There are many diets and biohacks out there, but the best one for you is the one that works for you. "Working for you" means:

1 - It's sustainable, in other words, you can do this for the rest of your life.
2 - It fits with your psychological preferences and desires.
3 - It works with your spiritual beliefs (i.e. vegans, Jewish customs, et).
4 - It works with your lifestyle.
5 - You enjoy it.

Then you can start optimizing things, which we will cover in the next chapter. The best way to optimize your results is to use "outcome-based decision making," or to guide your next steps based on your data.

It takes a fair bit of training and real-world experience to interpret the data and make the proper adjustments. This is where your coaches and Jedi council provide tremendous value.

The most valuable part of accountability is that your coach will see your data on a regular basis so that they can give you feedback on whether you're on the right track.

For example, when Matt hit a wall with his bodybuilding show prep, the right course of action could be a refeed and less training rather than a more aggressive caloric deficit and more cardio. An experienced coach can easily help you avoid these pitfalls.

A Jedi expert won't only know the theories, but also have real-world experience to apply it, which involves coaching psychology. A great coach is able to help you solve your emotional blocks, upgrade your mindset, and help remove your self-defeating beliefs.

Finding Your Jedi Masters

Working with a Jedi master involves investing your time, energy, and financial resources. You will also likely build long-term working relationships with them.

Here's a framework to seek out the best Jedi master and to get the most out of each working relationship with them.

1 - Have they cracked the code on what you're trying to achieve?

Seek out the coaches who have aced the goal you're trying to achieve in a reproducible manner. They should have a track record of success with someone like you.

A great Jedi expert should have real-world wisdom and insights beyond textbooks from having worked with many clients. Their expertise could be decades ahead of whatever's published in studies and books right now.

2 - Do you resonate with them psychologically?

Do you feel like you psychologically resonate with this person? Do you feel motivated by their communication style? Do you relate to them and feel like they understand you?

Some people do well with ass-kickers or bootcamp-style coaches who scream at them at the squat rack. Others do better with a more nurturing approach and need a lot of positive emotional reinforcement. The best coaches can change their style based on the person.

Specialists vs Generalists

Specialists know a lot about a little, whereas generalists know a little about a lot. If you need brain surgery, you definitely want a surgeon that is a true expert at that process.

Through the different phases in your life, you will need specialists to fix your problems. For example, at one time, Wade needed a bodybuilding coach. A few years later, he met Dr. O'Brien, a naturopathic doctor who helped optimize his digestion.

Specialists are experts at what they do, but there's one potential downside to be aware of. Specialists can be myopic and not be able to see the big picture accurately. For example, US medical schools teach, on average, less than 20 hours of nutrition education in their 4 years.[261] As a result, most conventional doctors know a lot about medicine and lifesaving procedures but very little about diet and a healthy lifestyle.

Some specialists also only give opinions or specific treatments they're trained to do rather than coach you through your health journey.

The one mistake people tend to make is that they tend to bounce from specialist to specialist. Sometimes, you will get conflicting information from two experts because they see reality from their specialist lens.

---

[261] Colino, S. (2016). *How Much Do Doctors Learn About Nutrition?*. Retrieved 2 October 2020, from https://health.usnews.com/wellness/food/articles/2016-12-07/how-much-do-doctors-learn-about-nutrition

In your Jedi council, you need at least one generalist who is a head coach or the master coordinator. They are the project manager for your health who integrates all the different moving parts. This person could be a health coach or an integrative or functional doctor. They can help piece together various points of view from different specialists.

Powermove: Find a Head Coach That Works for You

Your head coach helps you work on the right changes in the right order at the right times. They should also know many specialists so they can bring in the right experts at the right time.

Importantly, your head coach brings the data to life, helps reconcile conflicting data points and conflicting advice from different specialists. That way, you avoid being paralyzed by data. Instead, the data creates a motivating dopamine loop that drives you into action.

The head coach can also be an "offensive coach," who specializes in proactively reaching health, fitness, or performance goals. Or, they can be a "defensive coach," who specializes in preventive health and anti-aging.

Different Types of Experts to Include in Your Jedi Council

How To Choose A Great Generalist

The following section will help you choose and select a great "head coach" for your biological optimization journey.

Naturopathic Doctor

Naturopathic doctors serve different ideas that are not dependent on drugs. They usually have a wider array of knowledge in different areas.

Most naturopathic doctors are trained to be General Practitioners of natural medicine—they know a little bit about many natural healing traditions. Naturopathic treatment modalities can include herbal medicine, counseling, lifestyle medicine, nutrition, homeopathy, manual therapy, and traditional Chinese medicine.

Most accredited naturopathic colleges start off naturopathic doctors similarly to medical doctors. They learn the same basic and clinical sciences.

Like medical doctors, they perform physical exams, read labs, and diagnose both diseases and suboptimal health conditions.

However, naturopathic doctors are usually familiar with innovative labs that are not commonly used in conventional medicine. They can also help you with suboptimal health and disease prevention. Naturopathic doctors typically don't prescribe medications or perform surgeries.

Most of them go on to specialize in specific problems or populations. Each of them may also develop a preference for specific treatment modalities. Therefore, not all naturopathic doctors are created equal. A good naturopathic doctor can be a great head coach.

Functional and Precision Medicine Doctors

Many medical doctors nowadays recognize the shortfalls of conventional medicine. They also realize the benefits of nutrition, exercise, and other alternative healing modalities. Some call themselves "holistic" doctors.

Integrative medicine physicians are conventional medicine physicians (and in some cases, specialists or surgeons) with the conventional scope of practice but with an expanded toolbox. They support their patient's health holistically, treating their patient's mental as well as physical health. When necessary, they do prescribe medications and perform procedures.

Many integrative medicine doctors acquired postgraduate training in nutrition, supplementation, and herbal medicine. Others integrate their premedical backgrounds, such as fitness or herbalism. They may also partner with health coaches, nutritionists, personal trainers, therapists, or other types of practitioners.

Some integrative medicine physicians practice precision or personalized medicine. Generally, precision medicine relies more closely on biofeedback data and genetic test results. These doctors may use digital tools to monitor your data and adjust your treatments accordingly.

Functional medicine has very similar philosophies as integrative medicine. However, functional medicine is more focused on resolving the root causes of chronic diseases.

Because these fields of medicine are so new, most of these doctors practice on a cash payment basis rather than accepting insurance.

A progressive integrative doctor can be a great head coach for your Bioptimization journey.

Integrative Health Coaches

Another option to find your "head coach" is passionate health experts who are knowledgeable in a wide variety of health topics. We consider ourselves as part of that group. We are passionate about health, fitness, nutrition, biohacking, longevity, and brain optimization. This drives us to keep learning and making connections with other health experts.

This is why we have created the BiOptimization Coaching Program, you can learn more at: www.bioptimizers.com/coaching

Important Specialists for Your Jedi Council

The following section is a list of specialists that we believe are important for most people's goals.

General Practitioner Medical Doctor

Medical doctors are trained to treat diseases and save lives with pharmaceuticals and surgeries. They're important to have on your team because they can order any standardized lab tests that have been around for a long time. Doctors have the broadest scope of practice among all health professions. They can diagnose and treat diseases, and give you referrals to specialist medical doctors and other types of healthcare professionals.

If you prefer the natural approach first and to only use medications as the last resort, you may find conventional doctors of limited help. However, it is important to still have one on your team to monitor the conventional labs and medically monitor what you're doing.

We don't recommend relying 100% on a medical doctor. However, if you have been living on a Standard American Diet and lifestyle, the first step should be to visit your doctor for a checkup.

One of the biggest downsides of medical doctors is the significant gap between the latest science and breakthroughs and what they know. The medical system in general is usually a decade or two behind other health fields. They are slower to adopt new health modalities and wait for dozens of double-blind studies to undoubtedly prove something before they start using it.

Chinese Medicine Doctors

Traditional Chinese Medicine is a thousand-year-old healing philosophy that is outside the western framework. However, it is still very effective both acutely and long-term for issues that conventional medicine tends to fail.

Nutritionists

Nutritionists defer to their own biases. They may specialize in the ketogenic diet, vegetarian, Paleo, or the Food Pyramid based on what they're most aligned with.

We believe all diets work. THE DATA SHOWS ALL DIETS WORK. All roads can lead to Rome, but you can choose whether to go through the mountains. You have to decide for yourself which diet is ideal for you before seeking out an expert in the style of diet you're seeking to optimize. Ideally, you should find someone who's not stuck in one way versus the others, or at least understands that their favorite diet isn't for everyone.

Fitness Trainers and Athletic Coaches

We recommend working with a fitness trainer or coach who has been able to deliver replicable results with multiple people.

They come in a variety of specialties, such as whether you want to get back to the gym after an injury, prepare for a powerlifting meet, or get ripped and compete.

You want to pick one with the right psychology who can motivate you and keep you on track. Do you prefer ass-kickers who pump you up? Or someone who tries to help you resolve emotional blocks?

We are experts in exercise physiology, but we still work with exercise and movement coaches for the following two reasons:

1 - Accountability - It is easy for humans to default to the path of least resistance. If you know that you will get your body fat measured in about 2 weeks, then you will be more motivated because you know you're accountable for your actions.

2 - Exercise Form, which is the most underrated aspect of exercise. Matt once trained with bodybuilding champion, Ben Pakulski. He says, *"As a kinesiologist, I thought I understood form, but Ben managed to make me feel like an amateur. My back was sore for a week doing half the weight I normally lifted."*

   True for every type of athletic endeavor, most people learn bad habits and never become aware of them until they start working with a coach.

Chiropractors

Chiropractors aren't just someone who cracks your back. They can help you optimize structural components.

Nowadays, we live in a lifestyle that's very counterproductive for our bone structure and internal organ functions. Being out of alignment can stimulate the fight-flight-freeze response, creating unnecessary stress that affects your health.

Any minor postural issue can also cause problems up and down the kinetic chain. For example, if your back is off by a little bit, it can have ripple effects on other parts of the body, such as the hip, knees, and ankles. It can affect your gait and many other movements.

Chiropractors are not all created equal. For finding a good one, we suggest finding one that comes highly recommended by other people. In fact, a good chiro can be one of the innovative health professionals out there.

Soft Tissue and Manual Therapy Experts

You have three different types of soft tissues: fat (adipose), muscles, and organs. It's common to associate massages with muscular problems, but in fact, there are experts who manipulate these tissues, which can address different health needs. Being able to make use of these experts at the right time can have a profound impact on your health and metabolism.

Bodywork can be very beneficial as a stress relief and recovery tool, especially the gentler forms, such as Swedish massages. The skin on skin contact increases oxytocin (the hug hormone) while reducing stress hormones.[262] Massages can also activate the vagus nerve, which relaxes you and reduces inflammation.[263]

Some more intense bodyworks, such as Rolfing, deep stretching, and active release therapy are very beneficial to resolve tissue adhesion, promote recovery, and ensure that you move well. However, these types of bodywork can also be stressful, so if you already are under a lot of stress, these therapies may make it worse.

You can often find the best massage therapists either through referrals from people who have similar issues. If you work with a chiropractor, naturopathic doctor, or acupuncturist, they may already know a great massage therapist they can recommend.

---

[262] Morhenn, V., Beavin, L. E., & Zak, P. J. (2012). Massage increases oxytocin and reduces adrenocorticotropin hormone in humans. *Alternative therapies in health and medicine, 18*(6), 11–18. Available: https://www.ncbi.nlm.nih.gov/pubmed/23251939
[263] Lee, Y. H., Park, B. N., & Kim, S. H. (2011). The effects of heat and massage application on autonomic nervous system. *Yonsei medical journal, 52*(6), 982–989. https://doi.org/10.3349/ymj.2011.52.6.982

Physiotherapist

Physiotherapists (physiatrist) are medical professionals who diagnose and treat injuries, illnesses, surgical recovery, or disabilities. Their toolboxes may include exercises, manual therapy, and other treatment tools.

You may find tools and machines, such as the ultrasound and transcutaneous electrical nerve stimulation (TENS, or stim) in a physiotherapy office. They use these tools to support injury recovery, reduce local inflammation, and manage pain. A great physiotherapist should help you achieve a state of health and pain-free movement within a reasonable amount of time without becoming dependent on these machines.

Biohackers

Biohackers are an emerging new field of self-experimenters who leverage technologies, tests, devices, health practices, supplements, and procedures. Biohacking is the most technologically advanced world in health optimization.

Biohacking coaches are people who perform experiments on themselves. Biohackers are at the bleeding edge of science, to connect the gaps between what works best in reality and science.
Biohacking bypasses these lengthy processes so they can optimize their health, performance, and aesthetics much faster than formal scientific discoveries.

Keep in mind that many biohacks also come with potential risks because there is not a lot of clinical studies behind them. A good biohacking coach will advise you on ways to mitigate the risk and minimize side effects.

Nutrigenomic Experts

A nutrigenomic expert can recommend the right genetic test and interpret the results based on your clinical picture. Then, they make recommendations to optimize your genetic expression and address your genetic predispositions for a deficiency, disease, or a metabolic advantage. They can help identify weaknesses and challenges based on your unfavorable mutations, and advise you on how to address them.

Once you are aware of mutations and the potential challenges that come with certain diets, foods, substances, and drugs you can make adjustments because you are aware of it.

For example, if you have the slow version of the CYP1A2 gene, you are a slow caffeine metabolizer. Then, drinking three cups of coffee a day is probably not a good idea.

If you're genetically challenged for sleep, like Matt, then it's probably necessary to spend a lot of time, energy, and money to optimize your sleep.

Some of your genetic variants can indicate if you are more suited for a ketogenic diet, a high-carb low-fat diet, or a vegetarian diet, or whether you're built for fasting.

However, know that your genetics is not a life sentence. It is possible to switch on or off the expression of certain genes.

A nutrigenomics expert needs to be knowledgeable of genetics and epigenetics (the manipulation of your diet and environment to optimize your genes). But they also need to be able to put all the information into context and actionable instructions.

You have over 20,000 genes, so chances are if you try to go at it alone, you will be overwhelmed. A nutrigenomics expert will help you pinpoint which genes to work on or which supplements to take, in which order.

Ayurveda

Ayurveda in Sanskrit means "wisdom of life." It is an all-encompassing philosophy that has been practiced for thousands of years in India.

Ayurvedic practitioners classify body types into different doshas based on physiological and neurological parameters. Doshas also take into account vocation, temperament, body type, and diet.

Based on our experience, we find that ayurvedic medicine may be especially helpful for:

- Deep detoxification, such as with the Panchakarma practice

- Chronic metabolic conditions that don't respond to conventional medicine

- Learning about your life purpose and psychological tendencies related to work, career, and family life

Yoga Practitioners

Yoga means "union," or a spiritual practice that allows you to consciously be unified with everything in the physical and non-physical world.

One of the biggest benefits of yoga is that the slow meditative movement and breathing make it an exercise that promotes the parasympathetic nervous response. If you run on fight or flight or do a lot of hard workouts, you may find yin yoga very calming, restorative, and balancing.
The other key benefit is posture and stretching.

Powermoves:
Hire the Right Generalist and Practitioners for Your Goals

1 - Work with a generalist coach who can help you achieve your goals. They keep you accountable and navigate different tools, diets, and practitioners to get the result you want.

2 - Find practitioners who are highly recommended by people who have worked on similar goals as yours.